CANCER AND CONSCIOUSNESS

Barry Bryant

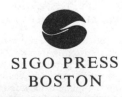

SIGO PRESS
BOSTON

SIGO PRESS
25 New Chardon Street, #8748
Boston, Massachusetts 02114

Publisher and Editor: Sisa Sternback

International Standard Book Number: 0-938434-73-X (cloth)
                                    0-938434-74-8 (paperback)

Library of Congress-in-Publication Data

Bryant Barry
    Cancer and consciousness / Barry Bryant.
        p.   cm.
    Includes bibliographical reference.
    1. Cancer—Alternative treatment. 2. Cancer—Psychological aspects
3. Medicine, Tibetan. I. Title.
RC 271.A62B78 1990
616.99'406—dc20   89-10755
                                               CIP

Printed in the United States of America.

Cancer and Consciousness

TABLE OF CONTENTS

Acknowledgments

My intention in writing *Cancer and Consciousness* has always been to stimulate dialogue between cancer patients and loved ones, patients and physicians, physicians and scientists, contributors and readers. Through a process of rich discussion and collaboration, I have been fortunate to exchange attitudes and feelings with people whose views you are about to read. I would like to express my gratitude for their participation in *Cancer and Consciousness* which I hope will be of benefit to many people.

During the ten-year process of working on this book, a great many people influenced me. Although their words have not be included here, they were very much a part of my personal consciousness throughout the process of writing. I would like to express my deep gratitude for their belief in and support of my work: Bob Applegarth, Elena Avram, Murry Baum, Bruce Bryant, Norvie Bullock, Tenzin Chonyi, Dr. Tenzin Chudrak, Terry Clifford, Ph.D., Marge Crespel, Melchia Crowne, Deschung Rinpoche, Dr. Yeshi Donden, Shakia Dorje, Professor Drakton, Dr. Lobsang Drolma, Dudjom Rinpoche, Donna Dudley, Russell Durgin, Dr. Ivan Gilbert, Dr. Mithlesh Govil, John Graff, Ea Hiss, Sam Holt, Peter Hujar, Ione, Kalu Rinpoche, Jamgon Kontrul Rinpoche, Dennis Konner, Esq., Dr. M.R. Kotwal, Helen Kritzler, Sidney Kritzler, Vivian Kuhrts, Dr. P.H. Kulkarni, Jerome Landau, Esq., Dr. Virginia Livingston, Jutte Marstrand, Barbara and Louis Marvin, Porter McCray, Linda Montano, Marvin Ostroff, Dr. M.P. Palange, Dr. M.H. Paranjape, Dr. Kenneth Pelletier, Erma Pounds, Sheldon Rochlin, Tony Romano, Elizabeth Selandia, Dr. Wolfgang Scheef, Holly Scheyer, Dr. John Schorr, Nathan Seril, Sharmar Rinpoche, Dr. C.T. Shen, Jing Shan Shiah, Beatrice

Smith, Diane Smith, Lobsang Samden Taklha, Namla Taklha, Geshe Lobsang Tarchin, Kathleen Conners Thetong, Tenzin Geyche Thetong, Tenzin Namgyal Thetong, Kenneth Thomasini, Jamphel Shenpen Ganden Tripa, Tempa Tsering, Dr. Phuntsok Wangyal.

Since January of 1983, my closest collaborator has been Maria Dolores Hajosy Benedetti. A gifted writer, editor and student of traditional medical systems, she has worked with enthusiasm and dedication on many aspects of this project, from transcription, copy editing, and correspondence to research and essential dialogue.

I would also like to offer special thanks to the following people whose input and editorial suggestions contributed so much to my own process: Mia Grosjean, Gregory Durgin, George Plimpton, William Myers, Marc Romano, Ellen Pearlman, Deborah Bergman, Stanley Carl Bryant, Lobsang Samten, Sarah Dudley, Ann Jones, Robyn Brentano, Nathaniel Scherill, my parents Carolyn and Frank Bryant, Pauline Oliveros, Judith Malina and Ilion Troya of the Living Theatre, Dr. Janet Gyatso, Patricia Zenn, Ann Wilson, Deborah Moldow, Ritty Burchfield, Eric and Janine Kuhrts, Toni Werbel, David Rosenthal, Frank Bryant, Jr., Dr. Carol Fleming, Carolyn Scheyer, Nancy Frame.

Special thanks to Samaya Foundation for continuous encouragement and the use of resources and facilities, including organizational and technical assistance.

"From the vantage point of space nations are not divided by lines or borders...people are not visible, but somehow the spell-binding, magnificent beauty of the earth seems to be indicative of the inherent beauty in all creation, which gives one hope that maybe one day we as humans will manifest that beauty in our relations with one another."

—Ronald McNair,
Challenger astronaut
10/21/50 - 1/28/86

INTENTION

This book is meant to be an ongoing exchange between each contributor and every reader. My intention is that *Cancer and Consciousness* will help people to create effective healing programs, congruent with inner beliefs and feelings about what will work best for them on an individual basis. Using the forms of healing we most trust, from diet, dreamwork and drawings to surgery, radiation and immunological drug therapies, we can become more in touch with our own instinctive abilities to heal and survive.

May this book stimulate deep thought, experiential knowledge, the making of meaningful choices, and always, more dialogue. And may this process of dialogue enable us to choose and create healing practices that nourish not only our minds and bodies, but also our communities and, ultimately, all life on our unique, oxygenated planet.

A special thanks to the contribution and dedication of my associate María Dolores Hajosy Benedetti.

Prologue

In 1979, my eldest brother Fred telephoned to say, "I have cancer...
but don't tell anyone."

Kinship With Cancer

Fred grew up the oldest of seven children in the town of Yakima,
Washington during the 1930s and 40s. At seventeen, during the Ko-
rean War, he joined the U.S. Marine Corps, where he served for
eight years, often travelling to far-away places.

In our early adult lives, we were separated by a generation gap
of sorts. As Fred was a "depression child" and I a "World War II
baby," raised in an atmosphere of relative affluence, our values, interests and ways of life differed greatly. In 1976, when I visited him
in the San Francisco bay area after almost twenty years of strained
communication, we came to a new understanding of one another
as we buried old hatchets and began to really listen to one another.
Our friendship grew, and his interest in my work and in the science
of meditation made for a growing bond between us.

Early in 1979 I found myself communicating regularly with family members regarding Fred's health. With recurring bouts of pneumonia, he was having a rough time trying to stabilize his normal
routine. One spring afternoon, as everything seemed to be coming
alive, the joyful sound of birdsong was interrupted by a phone call.
It was Fred, who ventured rather matter of factly, "I have lymphoma, a kind of cancer. Don't tell anyone, especially mom and dad."

In a state of utter shock I listened, and shaken, began to ask a
mountain of guarded questions: "How do you know? Are you cer-

tain? What did the doctor say? Is it a mild form of cancer?"

"It's treatable. My chances are good."

Having seen grandparents, aunts, uncles and some family friends suffer and die from cancer since my early teen years, the images that passed through my head were of gloom, slow mutilation and, in many cases, finally death.

Aware of his pain, and wanting to honor the confidence he'd shown me in sharing his secret, I struggled to answer his call for help. But even as I asked, "What could I do to help," not being prepared for this moment, I felt a sense of helplessness. What *could* I possible do? A queasy feeling of uncertainty worked its way through my body as our conversation filled with awkward pauses and silence.

Fred had always been a very private person, never sharing his inner thoughts or feelings. I was suddenly aware of how he'd overcome his emotional seclusion in choosing to share his very personal and terrifying news with me. With a sigh, I found myself torn between the anguish of his condition and the strength I drew from his confidence in me. Now, years later, I see that he had initiated a process of resolving long-term issues which would bring us closer together. This has helped me to see the undeniable karmic bonds of kinship which, in our day-to-day lives, take the form of family relationships.

As Fred and I talked that spring day, I heard our mother saying, as she so often had, "Our relationships are immortal." At that moment, I made a promise. "Fred," I said, "I'll be glad to start doing some research for you. I'll start reading and calling around to find out everything I can about lymphoma." I know that his response — "Could you please?... Maybe the Tibetan lamas know something... Pray for me..." — was for this very private man, a sign of healing on some level. Those were the words that empowered me to begin asking the questions which, in the ten years since then, have become *Cancer and Consciousness.*

During the weeks following Fred's secret disclosure to me, I began receiving mixed messages from family members. "He's feeling better." "We're not sure." "It's just pneumonia." "It's worse."

Aware of the social stigma associated with cancer, and concerned about Fred's fear, I decided to tell our parents of Fred's call, his denial and despair. Their response went beyond disbelief. "You're wrong... You're misinformed... It's not possible... He just has pneumonia. No."

"Mom, Dad, listen to me.... Fred called me to tell me he had cancer, and he swore me to secrecy. But the only way we can really help him is to be open and to accept this."

"No. Fred doesn't have cancer. No."

That long-distance telephone call left me in a state of suspension. I had to deal with tremendously strong but mixed emotions caused by being the bearer of bad news which my family wouldn't even accept. I knew that, to a great extent, their need to deny Fred's condition reflected part of our society's own "cancer syndrome."

Fred soon came to terms with his illness, and eventually told our parents of his condition. Several weeks after the "denial" phone call, I received a call from my mother, who spoke very matter-of-factly about Fred's cancer as though her denial had never existed.

Little by little, Fred became interested in making changes in his diet and behavior to complement his chemotherapy treatments. At about the same time, I learned that the great Buddhist teacher, Gyalwa Karmapa* of Tibet, also had cancer. He would soon be coming to North America for medical treatment, and to continue his teaching program.

Having been blessed with the opportunity to study meditation under the Karmapa's direction since 1975, I had experienced his warmth, compassion and great wisdom first-hand. I was eager to share what I had learned about cancer with him. During our discussion, I learned that Ea Hiss, a Danish-Tibetan Buddhist nun, had positively influenced the Karmapa's health with the Hippocrates Living Foods Diet.

Very impressed with Ea's work, I asked her to assist Fred with the Living Foods Diet while he underwent chemotherapy. Soon, all arrangements were made for her to spend six weeks getting Fred started. He was optimistic, and his wife Donna was very supportive. Results from the combined treatments were immediate and positive. His distended stomach diminished greatly. He was able to leave his bed, and resumed work with a vitality and lust for life that we had never seen in him before. During this time, the meaningful connection that Fred and I had begun to cultivate became stronger, and our desire to communicate cut through many old patterns which in the past had inhibited us both.

The entire family noticed a change in Fred's energy. He was exerting himself physically and mentally, and seemed fearless and full of the will to live. He used his new energy to begin to resolve much of what Elisabeth Kübler-Ross calls "unfinished business." This seemed to renew his appreciation for life in general. Seeing this new Fred, I was filled with questions and with surprise.

In the fall of 1980, Fred's business brought him to New York twice; each time he carried with him several vials of wheat grass juice. He

---

* For a discussion of the Gyalwa Karmapa and his relationship to this work, see appendix A.

would sit in my home for hours, in a state that seemed like peaceful acceptance of his condition and life in general. Admittedly, the diet, consisting of only raw, organic foods and a great amount of fresh juice, was difficult for him to adhere to. But he smiled as he told me that his strongest desire was to eat a New York bagel with cream cheese. During the next few months, he did gradually go off the diet, and his health was adversely affected.

During Thanksgiving weekend, Fred, Donna, and Fred's son Mark drove 500 miles south from their home in San José to my parents' place in Escondido, California, for a family celebration. The weekend went beautifully until the last moment. Then, without warning or apparent provocation, Fred attacked our father with a torrent of accusations and criticism. In his overwhelming need to release emotion, Fred was unaware of how much suffering his own suffering had caused.

Still in shock, a few days later, my mother called me in New York to tell me about the weekend and the incident. I heard myself saying, "Mom, you both have to forgive him.... It's part of the frustration, part of wanting to resolve old family business and not knowing how, part of the fear of dying, the uncertainty... it's part of the cancer." I tried to explain that Fred's explosion of anger had also served as a much-needed release — a purging, an expression of old emotions, even love for everyone. I reminded her of how he'd denied his condition at first. "Mom, he's in a lonely space. He's living with the cancer, and none of us are really prepared for being in life-threatening situations. None of us can really know what he's going through. Fred needs to find ways of trying to express years of repressed emotions. It's not so much what he's saying that's important; what counts is that he is able to trust us to help him relieve his pain." Then my brothers and sisters and I called our father to tell him of our love and support, and to let him know that Fred had only spoken from his own frustration, disillusion and fear.

It was a while before the debris from this crisis settled, but we all acknowledged that the turmoil had spurred us on to speak about many things which, for many reasons, had never been discussed or even acknowledged before.

Fred soon decided to move to Escondido, where, closer to our parents, he seemed to have everything he'd ever wanted: a large house on a corner, three businesses of his own. But his new life was a stressful one, and he'd gradually gone back to his old ways of eating meat, fatty foods, and refined, sugary products.

Even though he received chemotherapy treatments regularly, his health declined steadily and he thought only of preparing a secure future for Donna. He insisted that rather than focus on him, she concentrate primarily on their businesses. Donna was soon running all three of them singlehandedly. During the day she supervised two, and at night she ran the third, a telephone answering service, sleeping between calls. They spent very little time together, and despite hourly phone calls, communication between them was strained.

Upon my arrival at Fred's home on our last visit together, I was struck by an ethereal beauty that seemed to emanate from him. But a second glance told me that I was standing before a very sick man. We spent a week together, and he never once complained. He was very interested in me and my work. But as open as Fred and I were with one another, there were some things we did not discuss. The possibility of his actually dying was one of these. Instead, we focused on our joy at being together. Almost always peaceful, he expressed anger and anxiety only in relation to his inability to positively affect the businesses, a subject which he discussed only with Donna.

Meanwhile, in spite of the strain of their personal difficulties, Donna understood his condition, and offered much love and support. Although Fred had been estranged from the three children of his first marriage and the youngest child of his second marriage, he seemed to understand when his son Mark, the only child he'd raised and truly known, chose to leave him at this crucial time.

Two weeks before he died, Fred underwent a draining, unsuccessful surgery, even though six months earlier his own doctor had admitted that they were "driving in the dark without headlights." Then, two nights before his death, we spoke on the phone. For the first time, he made a demand of me: that I be in touch with our brother Frank, who had chosen to distance himself from the family for many years, and somehow get him to "make peace with our parents... to get all of us to realize the importance of having a good relationship with our parents... to work toward building harmonious relationships with one another." After we hung up, the phone lines blazed for hours as the entire family bridged the gaps, making peace. Fred's request was honored.

The following day, as Donna was preparing to take Fred to his scheduled chemotherapy appointment, he told her, "You know, I might die." Donna responded, "Yes, I know." On July 16, 1982 the doctor checked Fred in, confirming that the end was near. He died the next morning. My youngest brother Stanley and I flew from New York to join the others who had come from near and far to assemble at our parents' home for a special memorial.

Since our family had never been associated with any particular church or temple, we took this opportunity to create our own cere-

mony of remembrance, forgiveness and love. Spontaneously and
joyously, we all participated in making an altar of family icons and
photographs. It began with images of great grandparents and grandparents circling around a photo of Fred with mom and dad on either side, all surrounded by brothers, sisters, and his children. This
panoply of ancestry and youth was a meaningful reminder of how
each of us is part of life's unending cycle. Then sixteen family members sat in a large circle sharing poems, prayers, emotions and mem-
ories of Fred.

Fred's passing had brought us all together, and although *he* was
gone, Frank had come to be with us. As we went around the circle,
each of us spontaneously expressing a favorite story or memory of
Fred, Frank was the last to speak. His words opened a floodgate
of emotion which brought us closer together. The process of Fred's
illness and death had given us strength and allowed us all to feel
a unity that dissolved any personal differences.

On the plane, returning from Fred's memorial, I read a text by
the Dalai Lama on "turning adversity into one's ally," and spent hours
in contemplation. Although I had been greatly involved in a process of thinking, listening and talking about cancer throughout my
brother's illness, since his death my investigation took on even more
meaning. During that plane ride, I realized that all of my questions
about cancer, healing and dying—and the answers they had
elicited—were the beginning of a book of dialogue on cancer. This
is Fred's legacy.

INTRODUCTION

When I began researching cancer in 1979, the medical doctors I met with expressed frustration at a lack of progress in the field, but also expressed the hope that "a breakthrough is just around the corner." Several of the oncologists I spoke with seemed armored from the emotions of their patients. Although comfortable with their patients' technical questions, most of them were not prepared to offer desperately-needed psychological support to complement prescribed treatments.

Most of the cancer patients I spoke with seemed to see themselves as having few choices — most of which offered little hope. These people were struggling to find answers and direction while feeling hopeless, victimized, and isolated. I identified these feelings, along with the denial of illness and impending death (which I'd observed in my own family since childhood), as part of a "cancer syndrome."

The cancer syndrome brings with it a type of inner cold war, a moratorium on communication with our own bodies, an inability to hear the signals and messages coming to us from both physical and intuitive levels of our being. All too often, this syndrome makes a living hell out of the struggle to live. Because when we see ourselves as victims, alone, we lose sight of our innate ability to heal ourselves and one another.

When I began my investigation, I had two basic questions: "What is cancer?" and "How can we work together to understand its cause, prevention, effective treatment and psychological impact?" As I explored these ideas, my questions multiplied, and I was struck by a barrage of conflicting information which, instead of clarifying these issues, only confused me more.

In my desire to resolve conflicts and find "answers," I found myself dividing medical practice into two camps:"good," and "exploita-
tive" or "bad." This polarization helped me feel, somewhat
self-righteously, that I was at least narrowing down the field, and
moving toward finding "the answer." But dialogues with Tibetan lama
T'ai Situpa and Dr. Elisabeth Kübler-Ross awakened me to the fact
that I was involved in the same kind of closed-mindedness that I
so passionately criticized in medical practitioners. Thus, my polarized period ended abruptly. After my gentle confrontations with
these two teachers, I discarded almost all of the material I'd gathered
up to that time and began again, resolved to try and recognize the
beneficial aspects of all cancer treatments. During interviews, I began listening to people without the use of loaded questions, and for
the first time I experienced a nurturing, non-polarized dialogue which
helped me to see things in new ways. I also became more patient
with what seemed like little progress in the field of cancer treatment,
recognizing that each step, on every avenue, is part of human evolution and not just an isolated event.

What would help us go beyond the present models of seeing and
dealing with cancer? After long contemplation, I found the answer
through the act of writing this book. I had always been committed
to dialogue, but I suddenly saw that communication, the very process
of dialogue, was itself the essence of the solution I'd been seeking.

Of the many personal lessons I've learned, the most important
is about the importance of turning my fears into allies. Cancerphobia, a fear shared by millions (including professionals working on
the issue of cancer) taught me about internal dialogue, the need to
ask the "why's" of my fears, and to see them as potential teachers.
My fear has also caused me to think about how I would deal with
cancer, AIDS or any other life-threatening illness as a physical reality in my own life.

If catastrophic illness is to teach us, we must be willing to face
our terror of death and the fear of change with which we live on
a day-to-day level. Sharing our fears is a key to both recognizing
and dealing with them; dialogue is a means through which even
the terror may be transformed and/or released.

The ongoing exchange between scientists and health care workers who once would have considered themselves to be antagonists
within the field — even enemies — is dialogue in action. Complementary medicine, a movement toward meeting patients' needs through
varied approaches (ranging from homeopathy, creative visualization and diet to radiotherapy and chemotherapy), takes us beyond
the artificial barriers created by our collective fear. These methods

may be used simultaneously by patients desiring health care which involves their own participation in the process of healing on psychological, spiritual and physical levels.

Today, patients are more conscious of the need to learn about their medical condition and healing process. As they choose to obtain second opinions, get involved in personal networking and participate in support groups and other therapies, they activate and attest to the value of complementary medicine.

Because of my own background and experience, I've chosen to include three chapters related to aspects of Tibetan medicine, as well as a study of Tibetan medicine as an appendix. The Tibetan system is so different from our own that it demands that readers stretch their breadth of vision. Although it seems to have little in common with our modern system, like many medical traditions around the globe it is a perfectly valid, useful and time-proven healing science. Tibetan medicine is just one example of the many possibilities available to us as our world gets smaller and we become more interdependent

CANCER AND CONSCIOUSNESS

Understanding Complementary Medicine

MICHAEL LERNER, Ph.D.

Committed to raising the level of dialogue within the medical and scientific community, especially in relation to cancer, Michael Lerner, Ph.D. has been studying holistic healing models since the early 1970s. In 1981, he began researching and documenting complementary cancer therapies throughout Europe and America. He has met with several hundred medical practitioners, and has visited over thirty cancer-treatment centers. He has studied the work of England's Bristol Cancer Health Centre, Germany's Hans Nieper and Josef Issels, the Lukas Anthroposophical Klinik in Switzerland, and American practitioners including Carl and Stephanie Simonton, Stanislaw Burzynski, Harold Manner, Emanuel Revici, Michael Schachter, and many others.

A MacArthur Fellow, Dr. Lerner is on the scientific advisory board of the Institute for the Advancement of Health, and is president of Commonweal, a nonprofit corporation devoted to exploring aspects of health, education and human ecology. Commonweal is located in Bolinas, California.

In August, 1986, Commonweal's Cancer-Help program was awarded the Gertrude Enelow Foundation Award for excellence in humanistic medicine by the Association for Humanistic Psychology.

INTRODUCTION

In June of 1985, I traveled from New York City to Sonoma, California to videotape a three-day conference on cancer. As I taped a lecture, Dr. Michael Lerner approached me and introduced himself. When I explained that I was in the process of writing a book of dialogues about cancer, Michael—another "lay medical professional"—replied that he was involved in a similar research project. He and his wife, videographer Sharyle Patton, had even interviewed and videotaped some of the same people I had, plus dozens of others, in the process of studying complementary modes of cancer therapy.

I was struck by the similarity of our work and by the enormous amount of research he'd been able to do in a relatively short time. I was attracted to the possibility of learning from him, and in September I returned to California in order to meet with Dr. Lerner at Commonweal, where he has developed a center for health research, education and community service. The Commonweal Cancer-Help program enables cancer patients to learn about various approaches to cancer therapy and helps them to make informed choices in integrating the best of established and complementary approaches to cancer treatment.

Meeting Dr. Lerner and learning of his work supported my belief that attitudes which can help us understand cancer prevention and cure will come about through dialogue among medical professionals and lay people alike. Michael Lerner is committed to this dialogue, as he explores many approaches, perspectives and practices used in preventing and treating cancer.

DIALOGUE

BRYANT: Can you talk about your own personal motivation for working in the field of cancer research?

LERNER: I had long been interested in exploring complementary cancer therapies, and then in 1981, my father developed cancer. So the coincidence of my interest and my family reality brought me to study cancer more or less full-time.

BRYANT: Were you seeking out methods that your father might follow?

LERNER: I wanted to make the information available to him so that he could make any choice that made sense to him. I was not interested in pressing a specific alternative therapy upon him. In fact, I was somewhat skeptical that alternative cancer therapies would have much to offer. I'd been engaged in holistic health research for about ten years, and I was familiar with a general pattern of exaggerated claims in the field. When I started, I wasn't sure that *any* quality work was being done in alternative medicine. I was sympathetic to holistic therapies but I wasn't at all confident that they had much to offer to the cancer field.

BRYANT: How did your study evolve?

LERNER: I spent the better part of two years visiting thirty prominent individuals and centers in Europe and North America. I started out in Canada; then I went on to Los Angeles, San Diego and Mexico, and I visited virtually all the major centers in those areas. During that trip I saw a considerable number of cancer patients who had come down with essentially hopeless diagnoses, yet who reported that they were doing well. I began to feel that something was going on. Some results were being achieved.

I went from there to Europe, where I visited the major centers in England, Germany and Switzerland. That trip powerfully reinforced my feeling that some quality work was being done in the cancer field. The people and places in Europe that I found particularly interesting included the Bristol Cancer Health Centre in England, Hans Nieper and Josef Issels in Germany, and the Lukas Anthroposophical Klinik in Switzerland.

Then I came back to the United States, visited Emanuel Revici and Michael Schachter in New York, saw Carl and Stephanie Simonton and Stanislaw Burzynski in Texas, and went to the American International Hospital in Zion, Illinois, where I visited Harold

Manner.

Then I returned to San Francisco and began to learn more about the adjunctive cancer therapies, primarily the psychological therapies. All of this time, I was also speaking with numerous cancer patients and individual practitioners who are not too well known. My guess is that I spoke to several hundred practitioners and probably over a thousand patients in four years. And I've read a good deal.

BRYANT: Your work is an exploration of what you've come to call "complementary cancer therapies." Can you describe exactly what you mean by that term?

LERNER: I divide up cancer therapies this way: I speak of "established" cancer therapies, meaning chemotherapy, surgery and radiation. "Alternative" therapies are used in place of established cancer therapies. "Adjunctive" therapies are used along with established cancer therapies. I prefer the term "complementary" as a term that includes both alternative and adjunctive therapies, because their use varies so much. One can use "adjunctive" therapies alternatively, and one can use "alternative" therapies adjunctively. Both macrobiotic and Simonton therapies, for example, can be used adjunctively or alternatively.

I think the most important thing to say about all complementary therapies is that they encompass some of the best and worst practices in cancer therapy today. There are some great practitioners — ethical, thoughtful, compassionate people. There are also some true quacks. Both types can be found working in the field of complementary cancer therapies.

BRYANT: What do you look for in a cancer-treatment center?

LERNER: The places that interest me are places where, as far as I can see — and I do look carefully — the individuals involved are people of integrity. Second, the practitioners' theory about how their therapy works is coherent and plausible to an intelligent group of patients and other observers. Third, anecdotal reports show that some people have done well on these therapies.

BRYANT: Having examined many methods of cancer treatment, how do you plan to use the information you've collected?

LERNER: My interest is, very specifically, in raising the level of discourse about complementary cancer therapies. I am not at all involved in defending or recommending alternative cancer therapies over established therapies. My general view of complementary therapies is that one, there is no sure cure for cancer among the complementary therapies; two, there is very little scientific evidence with which to evaluate them; three, there is strong anecdotal evidence that people do well on many of them; four, many intelligent and resourceful people, who do not fit the caricature of desperate, credulous patients, are using these therapies; five, there is a strong convergence between the best thinking on some of the complementary therapies and some of the best thinking on established therapies.

That convergence, including psychological, attitudinal, nutritional and psychoneuroimmunological research straddles a very bitterly contested battlefield.

BRYANT: Where do you see yourself as fitting in there?

LERNER: Well, first of all, I'm not at all interested in the battlefield itself. I *am* interested in raising the level of discourse, and in supporting patients in making intelligent, grounded choices with plenty of information about how to create their own integral therapies — which may include established and/or complementary therapies.

I enjoy exceptionally good relationships with many members of the established medical community, not all of whom I agree with. I don't see it as my job to convince them of anything. I do want to encourage a more far-reaching dialogue.

BRYANT: So you would identify your own roles as researcher and reporter?

LERNER: Yes. My role is to serve as a social theorist and as a relatively objective reporter. I have a decade of experience in holistic health research and evaluation, with no axe to grind in this field. I do have a strong desire to share what I've learned.

BRYANT: In light of the five conclusions you've come to, what have you actually learned in terms of cause, prevention, treatment or control of cancer?

LERNER: Well, that's a huge subject, but prevention is the area that I feel most strongly about. There is awesome evidence of our capacity to diminish the major and least treatable cancers, especially through environmental and dietary changes. So I think that is where our major emphasis should be.

BRYANT: You say both diet and environmental factors.

LERNER: Yes. Take asbestos, for example — chemicals in the environment. Incidence of colon, prostate and breast cancer is dra-

matically less in Japan than in the U.S., and as Japanese people
emigrate to the United States, these rates go up. There is also strong
epidemiological evidence that improved diet controls cancer, heart
disease, diabetes, hypertension, and a whole range of chronic and
degenerative illnesses. America, in general, is moving very rapidly
in the direction of recognizing this. We, the American people, and
not the scientists, are taking care of these issues quite rapidly. Fighting environmental toxins is part of that. There is just an enormous
amount to be done.

BRYANT: And on the treatment side?

LERNER: I believe that a great deal can be done in cancer treatment. And it does not all have to do with *curing* cancer. It has to
do with *optimizing outcomes* for people with cancer.

Essentially, I believe that integral cancer therapies — those that
integrate established and complementary therapies according to
individual predilections and needs — are the real future of cancer
therapy in this country. And I think that you could also call these
integral cancer therapies "humanistic" cancer therapies, because
they basically give each person his or her best shot.

The emphasis is on empowering the individual cancer patient
to do what Dr. Larry LeShan calls "finding one's own song" at the
physical, mental, emotional and spiritual levels. That optimizes outcomes. And I think there is a describable strategy for doing that.

BRYANT: Can you describe this strategy?

LERNER: I frequently get calls from people — not the cancer patient, but a daughter or a son or a wife or a husband. And they're
all excited about complementary cancer therapies. They want me
not only to tell them which therapy their loved one should em-
bark upon, but also to convince this person to take that route.

My answer to those people is, "That's not how it works." The
struggle must be waged by the person who has the cancer. The
best thing you can do is to support that person in whatever he
or she chooses to do.

BRYANT: The choice of cancer therapy is a deeply personal
choice.

LERNER: Exactly. And nobody knows enough to tell someone
that his preferred way is the best way for someone else. In fact,
everything points to the fact that the people who do best — no matter what combination of therapies they may choose — have arrived
at their choice after looking at a wide range of possibilities. They've
chosen a therapy which makes the most sense to them; they've

been supported in this by their physician and their friends; and they've evolved as a function of their own desire to evolve. I think that's the key to the whole thing: supporting people in whatever they choose to do.

BRYANT: Besides being generally supportive, can you offer some guidelines for those who want to help someone in the process of choosing a system of cancer therapy?

LERNER: One of the problems I've observed is that people often spend less time deciding how they are going to treat their cancer than they would spend shopping for a new car.

The point is that people should recognize that there are awesomely different therapies and approaches to therapy, *even among established cancer treatments,* for the very same cancer. It's fine if you want to simply put yourself in the hands of a competent physician, assume that he has the information, and trust him. But you should be aware that there is an enormous range of approaches to treating cancer among established therapies, even within one hospital.

Of course, there is an equally enormous range of choices among complementary therapies. But the scientific data on complementary therapies is miniscule. It's helpful to characterize these therapies in categories like: nutritional, psychological, alternative immune, alternative use of established therapies, herbal, laying on of hands, spiritual therapies, and so on.

BRYANT: The process of choosing a type of treatment is intimidating to many people because, with the lack of scientific information on so many of the "alternative" methods, people really don't know what to base their choice on. And without the active support of their doctors, many patients feel overwhelmed. How do you recommend that a patient approach this kind of decision?

LERNER: It may be helpful to ask the following questions when choosing a system of cancer therapy: Does this means of health promotion work along lines of healing that make sense to me? If a therapy uses some particular symbolic substance as a "curative" agent, am I attracted to this route? Do I intuitively feel good about this symbolic process?

Because whether or not a method is effective, the placebo effect is one of the most powerful healing phenomena known to man.

The Institute for Noetic Sciences in Sausalito, California did an extensive summary of research that's been done on the placebo effect. A very substantial proportion of people tested in controlled, double-blind studies—placebo vs. active agents—report just as good results with the placebo in unleashing powerful healing processes. In fact, a full thirty percent of ordinary drug effects are placebo effects. So if you trust a particular medicine or therapy, there is ample scientific evidence that this will act as a very powerful healing agent for you.

BRYANT: It's important that each of us has a sense, then, of the immense breadth of choice in both established and complementary therapies. This understanding will allow people to choose ways that most closely reflect their own values and beliefs.

LERNER: Yes. I believe that the people who are primarily oriented toward established therapies should use those methods while being aware of complementary therapies which can be used as adjuncts. People who are oriented toward the complementary therapies owe it to themselves to find out what the established therapies can do for them. I've seen real tragedies because people have used complementary therapies while ignoring established therapies that would have given them years of additional time.

I tend to point toward a balanced approach. If someone is going in one direction, I say, "Fine, go that way, but look at the other." To me, an integral therapy is one that brings these two things together. I think this improves the conditions under which people choose whatever they regard as healing.

BRYANT: With all you have learned through your research, if you were confronted with the condition of having cancer, what kind of therapy program would you choose for yourself?

LERNER: I don't know. I think it would depend an awful lot on what the specific cancer was and what the conditions of my life were at that moment. And since I'm not actually facing that condition, my actual response is not accessible to me right now.

Certainly though, I do believe that it's important to work on the physical, psychological and spiritual levels at once. People who do best seem to work on all three levels.

In general, on the physical level, I would follow an energy-filled, vegetarian diet, without getting into a big hassle about the diet. I don't believe in hassling about any of these things a great deal. If you're drawn to a diet, work with it as much as it makes energetic sense for you to do that.

On the psychological level, I would work with a skilled counselor, and I might work as part of a group if there was a good group around.

On a spiritual level, I would recognize this as a very painful opportunity for personal growth and evolution. It's an opportunity to make the very best use of the time available.

BRYANT: It's reassuring, what you said about not hassling about diet. For so many people, working with diet does become difficult and complicated. Partially, I'm sure, it's because our dietary patterns are so very much entwined with our emotions—with old family patterns, with habits, and with what's culturally acceptable. It's difficult to give up the foods we've learned to associate with love and sharing, even if those foods are literally life-threatening. Can you talk more about your experience with diet?

LERNER: My father has experienced a long remission from a cancer after being told that he had only a very short period of time to live. But he never really cleaned up his diet. He did some symbolic things that were very important to him, such as not eating as much meat as he used to. But he never really changed his eating habits. He eats a lot of ice cream and other dairy products that he really likes, and he still drinks plenty of root beer.

Good diet is a choice that I would make—a choice that, in my own world view, is indispensable to the healing process. But there are folks out there who have turned their cancers around without touching their diet. If it's a real hassle to turn one's diet around and one isn't drawn to doing that, I wouldn't put too much emphasis on it.

BRYANT: Because the stress of changing one's diet could become more injurious than eating meat or whatever?

LERNER: Yes. That's the point. And since you don't know that it's going to work, you shouldn't do anything that is counter to what you want to do with the rest of your life. You should do what you want to do. Personally, I believe that turning diet around is one of the most powerful approaches to changing a cancer condition. But it simply isn't everyone's path.

I was talking with someone from the Bristol Clinic in England today who said that the Bristol attitude toward diet is changing. It used to be sort of didactic: here's our prescription for diet. Now it is: here are our suggestions for diet. The guidelines haven't changed, but the attitude is different.

People come to healing by different routes. Some people make good use of being totally meticulous with diet. They see the advantage; they see how they can make it work. Diet has tremendous placebo value for them, in addition to its biological value. So they get right into it. They become fanatics and purists about it, and they see great results. Other people are not drawn to that, but instead move toward the psychological work. Others are drawn to the spiritual work. Preferably one works on all three levels at once, but it doesn't have to be that way.

If something is really hard for someone, maybe that's not the right approach — unless that person feels, "Hey, this is really hard for me, but this is exactly what I need to do." Then, okay. Perfect.

BRYANT: Either during or as a result of your research and contact with cancer patients and treatment methods, have you experienced cancerphobia yourself?

LERNER: Oh, absolutely.

BRYANT: How have you dealt with it?

LERNER: With a lot of thought and a lot of prayer. In fact I would not say that I have vanquished it. I think it's part of our culture, and it's definitely part of my life. Having lived with it as a daily reality for years, it's less intense for me now. It seems to come up less often, but it's still around.

I'm aware of the fact that oncologists get cancer more than any other doctors — that the spouses of cancer patients die of cancer more often than other people. I think that's a risk you take if you focus a lot of energy on cancer in your life. I try to focus more on healing than on cancer. But if I do develop cancer through this work somehow, I don't think that it's the worst fate in the world.

BRYANT: If you were given the opportunity to speak at a symposium of doctors from the American Cancer Society or the National Cancer Institute, what would you advise them in terms of practices which might complement their administration of chemotherapy, surgery and radiation therapies?

LERNER: I have friends who work at the National Cancer Institute, and I have talked with a good number of physicians and oncologists. I recognize what a terribly difficult situation oncologists are in. I have a lot of empathy for them. It's a very tough job.

I think it's helpful for oncologists to recognize that there is a growing group of patients who want to explore the integration of complementary and established therapies. If established therapies have nothing to offer these people, it's useful for oncologists to recognize the strong scientific arguments which support the patients' choices. For instance, the complementary therapies in which these people believe are unlikely to harm them and may possibly be quite beneficial. These therapies may improve the quality of life and may even contribute to the extension of life. This is all very solid stuff. There are strong, credible arguments.

Familiarity with complementary therapies can only strengthen an oncologist's practice.

BRYANT: Similarly, if you were to address a group of medical educators, what would you suggest that they incorporate into their curriculum for future doctors?

LERNER: That's a really good area to think about. Young doctors in medical school should be offered a choice. Those who are not drawn at all to the humanistic aspects of medicine should be free to go forward and focus purely on the technical aspects of medicine. This is a perfectly legitimate route.

Others, who are strongly drawn to the humanistic aspects of medicine, will benefit greatly from our making the curriculum more humanistic. This is a very important objective, which is shared by the deans of many major medical schools in the U.S. today. They're really trying to do it. A lot is being written on the subject. Many medical schools, including Harvard, Yale and NYU, have organized complementary-medicine lectures and seminars. And I think this kind of thing is going to grow.

Ultimately, what's needed is a philosophical framework which enables established science to take its place alongside complementary approaches in a genuinely pluralistic medical system.

BRYANT: Would you say that patients themselves are responsible for much of the opening up and exchange of information that's taking place among professionals today?

LERNER: It's partly a function of patient demand, but historically, only about one or two patients out of ten are really interested in making the effort to heal themselves. Others can make small steps in that direction, but they're not really interested in a comprehensive healing program.

When Bernie Siegel started the Exceptional Cancer Patients Program in New Haven, he expected a lot of people to show up, and very few did. We offer similar programs at Commonweal, and I never expect people to break down the doors. It's like yoga or any other discipline. Not everyone is born to make that effort.

I'm not making a negative judgment. Most people simply have other objectives in life. They'll go to the doctor, wanting him to fix them as well as he can. If he can't fix them, they might prefer to do nothing rather than to try changing certain aspects of their lives. The experience of many people is that when they have attempted to make a major change, it hasn't been effective. In psychological terms, these people don't have what is called an inner locus of control.

Psychologists say that only about twenty percent of the population has an inner locus of control, enabling them to feel that what they do in life really influences outcomes in any major way. Siegel believes that those are the people who are willing to work on their healing processes through programs like the one he offers for exceptional cancer patients.

BRYANT: What would you say is the most important level of cancer-therapy development for the eighty percent who don't really want to participate in rigorous, complementary cancer-therapy programs?

LERNER: For eighty percent of the people, the really important changes in cancer therapy will be increased humanism in the application of therapies, and in the use of passive health-producing programs. That is, when they're in the hospital, the food will be a little better, the environment will be more humane, they might be introduced to deep relaxation and other things like that. Don't expect everyone to go home and use these things, but it's important to develop a system that offers high-motivation programs to those patients who do want to focus in that way—and then to be very compassionate.

Because the real tragedy of established therapy occurs when you've got patients who are going to die from a particular cancer, and chemotherapy is not doing them any good, but the physician continues to treat the tumor and not the patient. I think that approach is incorrect. It actually causes suffering, while there is a lot that could be done to diminish suffering.

BRYANT: We haven't really talked about psychological suffering or stress, which contributes to lowered physical resistance to disease, including cancer. What can you say about the relationship between stress and cancer?

LERNER: Stress research is a growing field. Research studies made on human beings show that stress greatly lowers resistance to the cancer process. Reduction of stress increases resistance.

For me it's easiest to talk about this in relation to my work with children who have learning and behavioral disorders. I was involved with them before I got involved with cancer.

I became convinced that learning and behavioral disorders in children are not an isolated phenomenon. They're just an example of increased biosocial casualty, resulting from the total environmental stress load on the American population.

If we look at the years since World War II, we see the nuclear revolution, the petrochemical revolution, the transformation of the American diet, the increase in both ionizing and non-ionizing radiation, increases in noise, crowding, and many other things.

During that same period, we see an increase in chronic disease at all levels of the population—increase in accidents, drug abuse, suicides among young people; increase of many forms of biosocial casualty.

The important thing to notice here is that in spite of all the problems—the stress, the casualties—not everyone has gotten sicker. In fact, some people have been getting healthier. And that's because there's more to the pattern than just increased stress causing an increase in biosocial problems. The evolution of individual health is related to patterns of both stress and nurture in the individual's environment.

Some things are intrinsically stressful, like chemicals at some levels, and noise. Many stresses, on the other hand, are a result of the individual's attitude toward the stress-identified factor. What might stress one person does not stress another, depending upon fundamentally differing attitudes. It's a very complex subject.

BRYANT: The stress factors you've mentioned are external ones, primarily.

LERNER: Yes. But, for example, yesterday I had an experience that illustrates one possible source of internal stress, and how attitude can change the potentially stressful experience. I had spent two or three days filling my computer with four articles I was working on, and then I dumped it all into the telephone for transmission to this office. Three of the four were swallowed by the computer, and I had no other copies of them. There's a frame of mind in which that could have been a very stressful event for me. But I chose to see it as an opportunity. I just felt, "This is not meant to be." Now there are times when I can't look at things just that way, and yet yesterday I could. That's the point about stress. I was able to transform and transcend a potentially stressful experience.

BRYANT: Sometimes it seems to me that our increased reliance on technology is causing the human race to evolve into two separate species. One gravitates toward more and more technology, and the other rejects technology and moves toward more natural ways of living. How can we facilitate communication between these two "schools" of being human?

LERNER: Your question assumes that I accept the premise that
we are, in fact, evolving in this way. I *do* accept the fact that balance is one of the primary issues of this age; and I believe it's also
the key issue behind your question. Some forms of technology are
beautiful and very elegant expressions of human potential. Here
I am sitting in a room filled with computers and high-tech stuff,
which play an important role in my life. But I devote my time to
working with natural systems of healing. The really important thing
to remember, first off, is that technology is a tool. It's an instrument in the service of human evolution, specifically in the service
of peace. And the conditions of peace are very similar to the conditions of healing. The ways we communicate with each other are,
at their best, ways that are conducive to peacemaking, both within and among people.

I'm influenced here by what Aldous Huxley termed the "peren-
nial philosophy." It encourages each individual to be aware of personal proclivities, resources and belief systems, and to find a special
path, appropriate to her or his own evolution. To me, that's really
solid. Because, whether personal evolution affects the cancer or
not—and I can't help but think that it does affect every illness to
some degree—personal evolution is personal growth. It's making
good use of our time.

Patient As Healer

BERNIE SIEGEL, M.D.

Bernie Siegel, M.D. is author of the bestselling book, Love, Medi-
cine and Miracles. *When the following dialogue was held, he was
active as a surgeon at Yale-New Haven Hospital, and as assistant clinical professor of surgery at the Yale University School of Medicine.
He is now an internationally-sought public speaker who has helped
to redefine the roles of both patient and physician.*

*As founder and facilitator of the Clinic for Exceptional Cancer
Patients, he also works closely with people who, while experiencing
cancer, AIDS, multiple sclerosis, and other diseases, are willing to
ask questions and take risks in the process of improving the quality
of their lives. Counseling, music, dream analysis, meditation techniques, picture-drawing analysis and, most basically, loving confrontation are the means he uses to help patients recognize and activate
their own role in the healing process. Dr. Bernie Siegel's second book,*
Peace, Love and Healing, *was published by Harper and Row in 1989.*

INTRODUCTION

In 1984, Elisabeth Kübler-Ross suggested that I meet with Dr. Bernie Siegel. I'd never heard of him before, but during the weeks which followed, Bernie Siegel's name and descriptions of his work seemed to pop up everywhere. Talking about him with others working to bridge the gap between purely mechanical and more fully integrated approaches to medicine, I was able to prepare for our discussion.

Our meeting took place in his office at Yale Medical Center of New Haven in January of 1985. As we talked, several doctors and nurses passed through the room to say, "Good night, Bernie." I couldn't help but notice a powerful note of respect underlying the informal phrasing. Dr. Siegel returned acknowledgment and love to each person, confirming all I had heard about him. I was impressed by the warmth and easygoing human exchange in what is one of the largest and most technologically sophisticated health-care facilities in the U.S.

As we talked, it became clear to me that established medical techniques were being administered here with a consciousness that each patient is more than just a complex of symptoms. Dr. Bernard Siegel is, in great part, responsible for this approach, and is committed to sharing what he has learned with the entire medical community—especially with those doctors who up to now have limited their work to the technological and mechanical aspects of medical practice.

DIALOGUE

BRYANT: In October, 1984 at the Inner Science Conference at Amherst College, I heard Dr. Kenneth Pelletier speak about the effect of mind on the immune system. His work involves research on meditation, biofeedback, and other means of altering the messages or vibrations that the body responds to.

Since then, more and more literature has been published in this field. Even *The New York Times* includes articles showing impressive results from psychoneuroimmunological experiments.

SIEGEL: There's been a tremendous breakthrough. Doctors and scientists all over are finding that we can actually program ourselves for recovery!

BRYANT: Can you talk about how this actually happens?

SIEGEL: Within the human body, information coming from our organs is transmitted to the brain, via the nervous system, in the form of vibrations. In every organ, there's a healthy vibration that reflects its "being in tune."

When something goes wrong, your kidney can't hold a sign up and say, "Help! I'm irritated. I need so and so." But its vibration, its message to the brain, changes. The healthy body will recognize this message. Then, if the correct directions are given, healing will take place.

BRYANT: It sounds as though you're describing an unconscious process.

SIEGEL: Yes, but the messages may also come to conscious awareness. The body and mind communicate through symbols. We can consciously interpret and benefit from the messages if we pay attention to the symbols. A dream or even a picture you've drawn may help to diagnose your illness.

I've had patients tell me, "I had a dream," or "An inner voice is telling me..." We may not know what's wrong on a conscious level, but on the unconscious level we always know exactly what's going on.

BRYANT: Why do relaxation techniques like meditation aid in the healing process?

SIEGEL: When we can calm people's fears and make them feel good, the body knows what to do. Peace of mind actually brings about chemical changes in the central nervous system. These changes induce recovery through the creation of harmony.

The actual techniques hardly matter at all. One doctor uses bio-feedback—I work with a picture-drawing technique, dream recall and other tools. Both of our patients get better because we're both helping the body respond to what I call the "Live!" message. We're both helping people to tune into their inner voices.

BRYANT: Can you describe the picture-drawing technique you use?

SIEGEL: First the patient is instructed as to the guidelines of drawing a self-portrait. Then, using all the colors, including black and white, each person draws: 1) him or herself, the disease, the treatment, and white blood cells combating the illness; 2) any scene or picture; 3) specific areas of concern: family, job, an operation; 4) other symbols such as trees, birds, boats.

Then together we observe whether or not the patient has deviated from certain norms. If so, we ask questions about those deviations, such as, "What does it mean to you, drawing yourself without a head, arms or legs?" These are the issues we look at: one's self-image, perhaps what the disease itself looks like, whether or not something is being denied. For instance, someone without a head, arms or legs would be showing himself as feeling helpless and hopeless.

One of the things you might do is to draw a picture of your family. Maybe everyone will be drawn without ears, showing that no one is listening to anyone else. We can observe how close the family members are to one another. It's a way of seeing what's happening. The symbolism helps you focus very carefully on the major source of trouble.

BRYANT: So, in effect, the drawing acts as a mirror.

SIEGEL: Certainly. One can't deny what one has produced. You can deny my interpretation, but the images are there.

BRYANT: The picture-drawing work seems like a time-efficient way to get in touch with a great deal of information.

SIEGEL: Yes. Quickness is important to a surgeon. I don't have much time to do this kind of therapy. And more importantly, the patient doesn't have much time in life to start spending hours in therapy. She may be dead in three months if she doesn't make some important changes.

The drawing works because it helps us see immediately: this is where you are today; these are the things that you have to change. It can really give you a sense of direction, toward the changes you can begin making now. *You simply can't remain the same person who got sick.*

BRYANT: How is your work with drawings related to the work you do with patients' dreams?

SIEGEL: In both cases, our goal is to convert information from the unconscious into consciousness so that we can take action. We can use our dreams to find warning symbols. The warnings always come. The information is always available. It's just a matter of knowing how to interpret the information.

BRYANT: The thing that strikes me as most amazing, and yet most natural, is that we all have the capacity to know *exactly* what is wrong, when something does go wrong. I think in most cases, we just don't have the confidence or the support we need to trust our own feelings. We're not used to listening to ourselves.

SIEGEL: Paying attention to our dreams is one way of getting in touch with ourselves. Martin Buber once said, "Revelation does not spring from the unconscious. It is master of the unconscious."

To me, dreaming lets us in on a spiritual, universal connection that tells us what we need to know and do. Reality isn't just when we're awake; it can also be when we're asleep, in touch with our true, divine connections and revelations.

If we pay attention to our dream state, then our awakened states will benefit by being more fully integrated and more beautiful. When we get up in the morning, we will know what to do all day and how to do it. Everything will seem better coordinated and organized.

Of course, we can deny our dreams, our feelings, and those inner voices. But without that closeness with ourselves, we'll miss out on living most fully.

BRYANT: I can see how the directness and honesty of your relationship with your patients must also help them to begin really listening to themselves and taking care of themselves.

SIEGEL: When we run out of tomorrows, we need relationships that can help mobilize the changes that must take place. An honest, loving confrontation with the situation is very often the most effective catalyst. I talk with people when they realize they might die soon. That's when they need it most; that's when they're most receptive, most open to change. It's no longer convenient to put off the changes they need to make.

In the process of making those psychological changes, the rest of the person is affected, sometimes dramatically so. The physical body may actually be taken care of as a side effect. In other words, when this person straightens his life out, his disease may straighten out too. The terminal patient may very well not die tomorrow.

BRYANT: Many doctors, when confronted with a terminal disease, hesitate to tell patients what they see for fear that the patient's despair will ruin his or her last days.

SIEGEL: There is no reason not to tell a patient what's wrong as long as hope is attached to the message. The patient knows exactly what is wrong inside. And the patient has the ability to deal with whatever is wrong.

BRYANT: It sounds as if you're trusting the patient's unconscious ability to diagnose more than you might trust more sophisticated, scientific means.

SIEGEL: The process I've described *is* scientific. It can be measured. It can be proven. And the ensuing healing process is also scientific — self-induced and scientific. There's nothing miraculous about it. It can be studied, and it is being studied as part of the field of psychoneuroimmunology.

BRYANT: Sometimes it's necessary to make changes in our lives in order for healing to occur. But our conditioning, old habits and attachments are strong and difficult to let go of. What about the patient's well-meaning family and friends, who may not like the changes suggested by you or another doctor? What suggestions do you have for patients dealing with interference or conflict at home or at work?

SIEGEL: We all have to learn to say yes when we mean yes, and no when we mean no — without guilt. You create your family. When you change, your family may reject and divorce you, or they may change along with you. There are a lot of options.

I won't let my patients become victims. If someone complains, "Oh, I could get better, but my family's a real problem," I'll say, "No, you're the problem. You created the family."

A simple example is the situation of a woman who is constantly being told by her husband that she's incapable of making decisions — that she's stupid. He constantly humiliates her for her inability to make decisions. When they're on their way to go out together, he even sends her into the house to fix her hair and change her clothes. And yet they run a real estate business where two million dollars will go through her hands in one deal.

The solution? When he comes home for dinner, say, "There's no dinner." "Why not?" "Well, you know I can't make decisions. I didn't know what to cook." When he asks, "Where are my clothes," she might reply, "I didn't know what detergent to buy. You know I can't make decisions, so I didn't buy any." And at some point then, he's going to stop bothering her. And she will regain the power she gave to him. She created the situation by allowing him to do that to her.

Or, as I said, she could walk out the door. On one hand, I believe that if you love enough, you could be married to the worst human being imaginable, and it would work. On the other hand, there may be elements that you really need to omit from your life to make things simpler and healthier. It may be necessary to divorce someone.

BRYANT: How do you deal with patients' fear of failure?

SIEGEL: I tell people that we have no failures; things are not good or bad. The issue isn't whether I live with my family or leave my family. It's what I do with either one of those options. How can I redirect energy that's not working for me? How can I learn to make it work in a positive way? What do we do with the pain we have? I try to get people to look at their pain without seeing themselves as victims.

I can't alter the world in order to make you happy or to "save" you. Only *you* can alter the world by changing *yourself*. I know the change can be scary. That's what really holds people back. Leaving a prison camp can be scary if you don't know what awaits you on the outside.

BRYANT: How does all the time you spend talking to patients and helping them deal with their feelings affect your actual work as a surgeon? Doesn't it cut into your medical practice?

SIEGEL: The sharing doesn't take away from my practice. It *is* my practice! Shouting at everyone, "I'm a busy man! I don't have time for your questions," helps destroy people. And I've seen that happen.

It does take longer to talk to people. All the talking to people I do adds up to an extra hour or so in the office each day, but everyone leaves happy. The other way, you end up leaving half an hour early, and everyone is unhappier after having seen you than they were before they came—including you. Because if a doctor keeps saying, "I'm a busy man. Talk to my nurse," that person cuts off not only his patients, but also himself.

BRYANT: And yet many doctors practice as if their attitudes don't matter—as if only the drugs they recommend really matter.

SIEGEL: One reason for that is the fact that we do have some remarkable substances, which we call "magic bullets." These drugs work without any reliance on people's belief systems. Their efficiency has nothing to do with the placebo effect. Take penicillin. If I can prescribe penicillin, I don't have to ask you what happened in your life last week, or why you're run down and tired. And the more miracle drugs we have, the easier it is to forget people's own self-healing ability.

BRYANT: So our dependence on miracle drugs may actually distract us somewhat from our natural healing potential.

SIEGEL: Meanwhile, cancers have actually gone away after people have been given injections of water, thinking they were getting some wonderful new drug. That isn't looked at in the medical profession. No one says, "Look, I want you to know how powerful patients are. If you tell them they're getting a wonderful new drug, they can get better with just water. People can stimulate their own immune systems."

Doctors aren't taught this. They're taught instead, "Here are the drugs. Give them to people. If these drugs don't work, they're in trouble." So we don't bring out people's natural healing tendencies. The drugs we learn to respect and depend on don't rely on people's active participation.

Now the drugs do work, and surgery works. Radiation works. And we should all strive to excel at the mechanical aspects of healing. But the truth is, if you want the best results, and you want to get someone well who isn't "supposed" to get well, you ask that patient to work *with* you. Then you've got everything working for you. And you'll see results. It's as simple as that.

BRYANT: You don't seem to be pitting the alternative-medicine movement against the established allopathic medical system.

SIEGEL: Some people think that the established medical system is in direct opposition to the alternative medical movement. But we wouldn't need alternatives if a lot of the things I've described were practiced more often. Mostly it's a loving attitude, caring for your patients. People respond to that. And nobody really knows then whether it's the treatment or the patient's own ability to heal that turns a condition around. When one's central nervous system "believes" that surgery is going to be a healing experience, a patient wakes up, doesn't have any pain, says, "I'm a little sore, but thanks very much," and is out of the hospital in just half the time.

BRYANT: You're very optimistic. Some would accuse you of spreading false hope.

SIEGEL: The concept of false hope is one of the most ridiculous things I know of. I ask students to give a definition of false hope. A "correct" answer would be, "Telling a patient he can live, when ninety percent of the people with that condition die." Phooey! Why should we try to authorize hope according to the statistics? Hope is the variable that can *change* the statistics.

If only ninety percent die of a condition, then let's stress the fact that that person has a chance of not dying. If you tell a group of those people that they are the ten percent who will survive, you may find that thirty percent or forty percent or fifty percent get better.

The professionals make a real mistake, saying, "I don't want to give you false hope. Nine out of ten people with this condition die of it, so you're probably going to die." With that kind of outlook, you're likely to have less than a ten percent survival rate, because everyone gets depressed, and some say, "Why should I even go through all the treatment if I'm going to die of this thing anyway?"

These are questions the profession has to deal with: What is false hope? What is truth? How do you talk to people? What is detached concern versus rational caring?

BRYANT: In general, you're helping people to work with attitude, and to improve the quality of their lives. Yet you're not espousing any particular regime to follow. You don't seem to be promoting any particular means of doing this.

SIEGEL: It's a very simple process. No exclusive or elaborate techniques are needed. Even television or radio can be a tremendous source of relaxation if it's set up for laughs, or for educational or meditation programs. Anything that helps the patient to relax is healing.

BRYANT: The best part is that this process of healing relaxation is accessible to everyone.

SIEGEL: Yes. And it's tremendously important that healing be recognized as something which is done *by the patient*, something which is *not an accident*.

BRYANT: So many doctors are losing their patients to cancer. They're having to deal with tremendous feelings of failure.

SIEGEL: Many of us feel like failures because our patients die. But obviously, anyone whose goal is to help someone else live forever will be a failure. "Not letting them die" is the goal of too many doctors.

On the other hand, someone who is working to help change his patients' life can be a total success, no matter how long that new life lasts. Living forever is not our goal. Improving the quality of life is.

BRYANT: Can you talk more about the people you call exceptional cancer patients?

SIEGEL: The exceptional patient is willing to fully participate. And it's surprising to find out how very few people choose to take on the responsibility of their own healing process.

Most people are waiting for a mechanic to come and do something: "Give me a pill, operate, do something." Only about one fifth will say, "I want to participate. I want to help myself." These are exceptional people. They are willing to deal with the pain of their lives in order to help themselves. They have a great deal to teach us about how to survive, and how to live.

BRYANT: These exceptional patients go largely unnoticed by the media, so they're an important but mostly unrecognized minority.

SIEGEL: Yes. It's just too bad that they *are* the minority. Instead of being respected by the medical profession, these patients are called pests and nuisances, because they are assertive and communicative and want to participate. Eight out of ten people that I see are not like that, and the remaining two are most often put down by other doctors: "Why are you asking so many questions? Why are you so eager to participate? Why are you upset? Why do you need to see your x-rays?" They're called "uncooperative patients," or "poor patients." Ironically, studies have been done to show that these "poor patients" are actually long-term survivors.

So it's totally backwards, you see. The "good" patients do exactly what the doctor wants them to do. Meanwhile, "bad" patients have the best chance of survival.

BRYANT: So you seek out these non-conforming "bad" patients who resist the system.

SIEGEL: Right. They're willing to look at the total picture of their lives. They're not afraid to examine or share their feelings, and they're not afraid to change.

If we change enough we can reject sickness, because it belongs to the "old" us, and we are a new person. Not that it's an easy thing to do. W.H. Auden said,

> We would rather be ruined than changed
> We would rather die in our dread
> Than climb the cross of the moment and
> Let our illusions die.

In many cases it's far more painful to change a part of your life that's making you sick than it is to undergo surgery.

BRYANT: And yet the changes we make to heal our bodies and/or to come to grips with an emotional problem may actually be changes needed by our whole selves. Do you think this is how "spontaneous healing" occurs?

SIEGEL: The spontaneous-healing response probably has something to do with the body's finally recognizing that it has cancer and then destroying it. Because the only thing that can reverse the cancer's progress is a strong immune-system response.

If we introduce an animal's organ into your body, your body recognizes that it's foreign, and attacks it. If we can get your body to recognize a cancer as foreign and attack it, that would be wonderful. But too often, the cancer cells aren't recognized because they're so similar to the body's healthy cells.

In self-induced healing, changes within the individual are mediated through the immune system. And immune globulins, "natural killer cells," are activated by outside influences like attitude and lifestyle. Changes of lifestyle and attitude, a new joy in living, learning to love, and the resolution of conflicts all activate the immune system to overcome disease.

BRYANT: You make it sound like the most natural thing in the world, but spontaneous healing is most often presented as a miraculous, isolated event.

SIEGEL: Spontaneous healing is a lot more common than we generally acknowledge, but it is not common for physicians to hear about it—because when people get well when they're not supposed to, they're not likely to come to a doctor's office. Why sit in a waiting room and pay lots of money if your disease is gone?

BRYANT: Do you think that spontaneous healing is something we can teach ourselves?

SIEGEL: I happen to believe that this process of healing can be taught. There's no tried and true method, of course, and it's not for people who are going to feel like a failure if the disease doesn't vanish. But if you want to participate, there are some things you can work on and try to do.

BRYANT: Can you talk about some of the scientific experiments that have been done investigating spontaneous healing or immune-system stimulation?

SIEGEL: Experiments have been done showing a movie, for instance, of Mother Teresa doing charitable work, and the immune globulins of viewers are actually strengthened during that time. By the same token, we try to reprogram a person's immune-system response by changing how he or she lives, increasing the "Live!" messages. The killers are depression and despair. And stress causes a lot of people to lean toward despair, which suppresses their immune system's function.

For instance, it's been shown that when you lose a spouse, the incidence of heart attack, infection or cancer is much higher. The immune system is suppressed because of the loss and because of despair. So when you teach people to survive, you're working through the immune system.

BRYANT: In most physiology and biology classes, we learn that the nervous system and the immune system are independent of one another.

SIEGEL: Now we're seeing more and more that the nervous system and the immune system are really one unit. They're not two separate things.

If we look at the year or two before an illness, ninety percent of your patients will be able to tell you very simply about some significant life change. And most of the time it will have been some kind of loss: anything from retirement to a death to a move. But "change" is a better word to use than "loss," because not all of these catalysts seem like negative events.

It's interesting that even events which might seem quite positive—a better job, a move to a new community, having a baby—may all cause a certain amount of shock, and may all trigger illness. It has to do with one's ability to deal with stress. Then again, we each get the disease we're programmed for by our personality, upbringing and exposures. So while I'm talking about just one event—a loss—disease has to do with the many factors involved in who we are and what we're like. Personality plays a large part in predisposing certain parts of our bodies to illness.

BRYANT: And the immune system responds directly to our state of mind?

SIEGEL: I think the immune system does respond to both feelings and images. Certainly, depression can make you sick. Depression can kill you. On the other hand, if you live and love and laugh, you'll probably have about a tenth of the problems other people have.

In terms of images, you can simply picture things happening in your body, and your body responds to these pictures. You can even talk to your body and it will listen.

BRYANT: You support the idea that health is a state of harmony on many levels. The problem is that many of these levels are not understood and so are ignored by standard medical practitioners. Why? What do you see as being primarily responsible for medicine's current inability to see "the whole patient?"

SIEGEL: I think it has to do with the way we're trained. In medical school, you're taught things like "detached concern," which is an absurdity. You can't be detached and concerned at once. I think that what they may be meaning to say is, "Don't act like a family member and get overly emotional." Fine. But that doesn't mean I shouldn't have any emotion—that I can't give my patient a hug—because that hug can make the patient *and me* feel damn good.

Everything is depersonalized, so we're talking about gallbladders, not people. You become a mechanical entity. There's no reason we can't be tender and caring while dealing with all the facts we've memorized. But we're not taught to harmonize these two aspects of medical practice. We're expected to function devoid of humanness. You end up treating diseases and entities, not people.

BRYANT: Do you foresee medical students becoming more sensitive to patients' personal needs?

SIEGEL: The questions I ask my medical students in order to wake them up are, "What did you learn in your course on healing?" Answer: "We don't have one." "What did you learn in your course in how to talk to people?" Answer: "We don't have one." What did you learn in your course on dreams and images?" "We don't have one." I think these are things that need to be looked at, because doctors don't know why they became doctors, or what their own fears are. They don't know how to talk to people to give them hope. All these things need to be integrated. Slowly, both students and patients are beginning to speak up.

If in medical school they said, "We need to know all these facts, but the important thing to remember is that this is happening to a person," it would help a lot. But we don't. And we don't look at issues. We don't ask why people get sick when they do—why people get well when they do. We don't say, "What's going on in your life?" That's not a question that medical students are told to ask anybody. Instead we ask, "Did your father ever have diabetes? Have you ever had this or that?" The time relationships are not made. We may find out that your husband died, but we don't ask whether it was three weeks ago or two years or ten years ago. Often you'll see facts in a chart, but few people learn to connect those facts to the lifestyle of an individual."

BRYANT: How do you visualize the future of medicine in the West?

SIEGEL: I think much more attention will be paid to dealing with individual patients as people — to the whole and entire process of healing. The system is changing, and I think Western medicine will become more of a healing profession than it is now.

On the other hand, I think you have to be a damn good mechanic before you do the other things we've been discussing. Spirituality and love may not be enough to save your body if you've just undergone poor surgery.

BRYANT: Practically speaking, as a surgeon, is there a difference between the way you operate and the way another doctor might approach a similar operation?

SIEGEL: My surgical practice doesn't differ from the surgical practice of my colleagues, although I think you'd find the atmosphere in the operating room quite different. I try to make it a healing experience. I hold hands and talk with patients when they go to sleep, and do the same thing when they're waking up. I play music during the operation. We know patients hear us during surgery, so I try to include the patient as part of the team. I talk to the patient throughout the procedure, sending positive messages, telling about what we're finding. That's so that they don't wake up having heard a lot of negative messages from which, under anesthesia, they couldn't defend themselves.

Even if people don't have anything positive to say in the operating room, I tell them, "Don't say anything negative. Say nothing rather than be negative."

BRYANT: Can playing music be a distraction to the staff?

SIEGEL: No, the music is not to drown things out or distract us. If anything, I'm trying to remind people that we're working on a human being. I might ask a patient what he or she would like to hear, but mostly I play spiritual music, because I want to bring the spiritual back into the operating room.

Research shows that patients with rooms where they can see

the sky heal faster than patients facing a courtyard. So part of what we're trying to do is to help connect with that vision again.

BRYANT: How did you come to work with cancer patients?

SIEGEL: I came to this work accidentally, in a sense. As a surgeon, cancer is simply the most threatening thing that my patients have to deal with.

Personally, though, my evolution as a physician comes directly out of the pain I experienced being unhappy as a doctor. I was uncomfortable with the mechanical approach that we were taught in medical school.

BRYANT: How were you able to get in touch with some of your own pain that you faced as a physician?

SIEGEL: The solution really came through workshops like Elisabeth Kübler-Ross'. They were a great education to me. They helped me learn how to be a good doctor. They helped me get in touch with the futility of having learned only to be a mechanic and a lifesaver.

BRYANT: So you had learned to depend only on your technical skills.

SIEGEL: Yes. That's part of it. There was also the fact that as a doctor, you're allowed to touch people, but only in a mechanical way. You don't say, "Here's a hug." You don't say, "I could cry along with you," or "I love you," or "I care about you." You have nothing to do if you can't help them mechanically. You're only useful as a saver of lives.

Let's say you come in and I operate on you. My success is measured by whether or not I saved your life. If I can't save your life, I'm a failure. That was my pain, and my catalyst. I was mostly motivated by the fact that as a doctor I didn't have a satisfying role. But now I don't feel like a failure, because I can help you to live. After all, you're not going to live forever, no matter what I do.

Maybe someday you'll even walk into my office and say, "Thank you for teaching me how to live and how to love. This is changing my life." Because, whether you're cured of your illness or not, you've learned something about how to live. This is the part of my work that really makes me happy. By teaching people how they might live more fully, I feel I'm giving more to the world.

Part of my role is still a mechanical one, which is fine. There's nothing wrong with my taking out your appendix or excising your cancer. But in the larger context, my work has to do with helping you go on from there.

BRYANT: Part of your evolution as a physician must have involved dealing with some of your macho male conditioning. You've obviously come to embrace the soft and nurturing aspects of your nature.

SIEGEL: Yes. We're talking about a balance between an ability to be assertive in making informed decisions about people's lives, and an ability to recognize and share feelings. I encourage my patients to show emotion without saying, "Be strong." I let them get angry. When they do, I say, "Great. Wonderful. You're a survivor." That can turn the anger around. I'm telling them that what they're feeling inside is perfectly all right.

It's not a formula. It's not saying, "Don't do this. Don't do that." More than anything, it's a matter of loving people. Only through love does someone realize that he or she is lovable. Only then can that person begin to throw off the old messages and forgive their parents and all the other people who've "screwed them up."

BRYANT: In your own practice, you've had tremendous success focusing on patients' strengths and needs as much as on their actual health problems. What do you think it will take on the part of doctors and patients before that approach is adopted on a wide scale?

SIEGEL: I think it will take a redirection of the entire medical profession. Right now we're just trying to keep people from dying— transplanting organs technically, and on and on. To me that gets to be absurd. I think the medical profession has to redefine what it's here for, which should be, in my mind, to alleviate suffering and to give more love to the world.

BRYANT: Do you think that this redefinition of the medical profession will come about through increased pressure from patients, primarily?

SIEGEL: I think that the pressure will be coming from patients, students, and to some extent, from within the profession. We're asking, "What is life? What is death?" and these issues are coming up for everyone.

One of the problems right now is that for many people, "M.D." stands for medical deity. This makes it difficult for most physicians to really deal with other human beings openly and honestly, because the "doctor" in your name helps you hide behind your status. You don't have to really deal with feelings. It seems easiest to play that role. I think we have to start producing a different kind of physician, one who is not afraid to deal with his or her feelings—

especially the pain.

Too many doctors are depressed because they only see their failures. Every doctor should have an annual party for all his patients who got well. That would really help change his attitude toward all the people he sees that year. One of the things you're not taught in medical school is that your patients can restore you. And yet patients are our greatest resource.

You can be an oncologist, take your sickest patient, the one who may be dead in a day, and say, "I need a hug today. I'm having a hell of a day." That patient will reach out and give you a hug, so that the patient can become your own therapist. He heals you in the process.

Without getting this sort of feedback, all you know is that everyone has cancer; everybody dies. And it just wears you out.

BRYANT: What can you tell doctors who want to relieve some of the frustration—who want to establish better relationships with their patients?

SIEGEL: We've all got to share our pain. That's the simplest answer. Honest communication. Sharing our pain is the way to get better.

A Biological Approach to Cancer Treatment

DR. CHRISTIAN KELLERSMANN

Dr. Christian Kellersmann is active as a naturopathic and homeopathic medical practitioner in Bonn, West Germany. A member of the European "biological" school of physicians, he specializes in using plant-derived and other nature-based medical preparations. Dr. Kellersmann, who holds a Ph.D. in holistic medical philosophy and various medical degrees, has written many articles on cancer prevention and control, and has lectured extensively on cancer and other aspects of health, including environmental factors and nutrition. President of the International Federation of Health Practitioners, he is an expert on naturopathic practices. In this capacity, he is presently advisor to the Minister of Health of the Federal Republic of Germany. He has also served as advisor to the President of Pakistan, the Minister for Health of Pakistan, and the National Institute of Health of Pakistan.

INTRODUCTION

Dr. Kellersmann was the first physician I interviewed for *Cancer and Consciousness*. Very much a teacher, he generously offered me an intensive course in biology along with many valuable insights, which allowed me to pursue subsequent interviews with awareness and confidence.

Much like Marshall McLuhan of the 1960s, who examined U.S. media through his Canadian "window," Christian Kellersmann and others living beyond our borders have the ability and vision to observe the U.S. cancer-care community through their own special windows. From these vantage points, able to perceive both the strengths and weaknesses of our advanced technological practices, they offer us perspectives that may help us go beyond current limitations.

DIALOGUE

BRYANT: Dr. Kellersmann, according to your own training and experience, exactly what is cancer, and how does it originate in the body?

KELLERSMANN: Ideally, every cell of every organ is genetically programmed to contribute to the perfect formation of that organ, and of the body. Normally, when a particular organ reaches its ideal, predetermined size and form, its cells stop multiplying. However, if the genetic programming of those cells has been disturbed through irritation, toxic exposure or other factors, including psychological ones, the disturbed cells may reproduce in an uncontrolled fashion. This may result in a cancerous mass, which could double and redouble in size during a short period of time. The mass itself robs the body of space, energy and nourishment.

BRYANT: So cancer functions parasitically.

KELLERSMANN: You might say that it functions as a parasite, but it's an *iso*parasite. That is, it originates from the body's own cells, and is not the result of an invading, outside force like a virus.

BRYANT: Is there a stage during which cancer is particularly dangerous?

KELLERSMANN: Yes. Death most often results when somehow these cells spread beyond their original, contained site. The spreading process is called metastasis, and it's extremely difficult to control once it's begun.

BRYANT: Are tumor cells actually healthy enough to compete with normal cells?

KELLERSMANN: Yes. Tumor cells, in general, are quite vigorous. They differ from other cells only in that they harm the body rather than help it, using the body's energy without rendering a service.

BRYANT: How does a relatively healthy body keep from getting cancer?

KELLERSMANN: In the healthy body, phagocytic white blood cells are programmed to devour invading organisms or mutant cells. These "killer" cells are being produced constantly by the body, and are a natural guardian force against cancer cells and other invaders.

BRYANT: So cancer cells are mutant cells which for some reason are not being destroyed by white blood cells?

KELLERSMANN: Yes. Nature is constantly producing mutated cells and organisms, which are present at some time in all of our bodies. But the healthy body's genetic instruction is to eliminate these cells. *Cancer only results when the immune system's eliminatory process has been disturbed or weakened.* For this and for many other reasons, it seems to me that the real issue at the close of the twentieth century is the strengthening and support of the immune system. We must learn how the immune system becomes weakened, and how we can support it or otherwise prevent it from becoming weakened.

BRYANT: You mentioned that the body's normal immune response may be weakened through irritation or toxic exposure. Can you say more about that?

KELLERSMANN: Cancer often appears in places which are exposed to constant irritation. Although this irritation may not be the cause of cancer, it certainly is associated with the location of cancerous growths. For instance, gallbladder cancer occurs most frequently in people who have had an irritating gallstone. Lung cancer appears most often in the bodies of people who irritate their lungs with cigarette smoke and other airborne substances. IUD users, who are exposed to constant uterine irritation, are more likely to get cancer of the cervix or uterus than other women. Of course more common, modern irritants such as the pollutants in the air we breathe, even the highly processed, chemicalized foods we eat, affect our susceptibility to cancer. And of course we all know that radiation spurs cancer growth.

BRYANT: Most of the irritants you've mentioned seem to be associated with modern life. Would you say that cancer is a disease of modern, civilized people?

KELLERSMANN: Cancer is not a new ailment. Cardinal Richelieu of the eighteenth century seems to have had cancer. According to historical records, he once had to be carried from Rome to Paris on a bed. He couldn't sit anymore; he was all swollen up and couldn't defecate. This indicates cancer of the colon.

BRYANT: But you can hardly compare one case of cancer two hundred years ago with the widespread incidence of cancer today.

KELLERSMANN: No, of course not. For many reasons. Today, we are forced to breathe chemically polluted air. We drink treated water. We eat processed foods which are low on vital nutrition and often loaded with chemicals. We get little physical activity.

Also, although discoveries and widespread acceptance of modern sanitation practices have probably helped to prolong human life more than any other modern medical discovery, our downfall today may actually have something to do with the fact that our sanitary standards have become almost "too perfect."

For instance, most health professionals today tend to rely far more heavily on quick-acting antibiotics and cortisone preparations instead of doing the natural thing: building up the immune system so that it is more able to produce antibodies. Because of the quick results and the convenience antibiotics offer us, we favor them, although they actually weaken the body's ability to fight disease.

Ignoring our own antibodies in favor of drugs we have invented to take their place is extremely foolish. We should build up our immune systems and not be dependent upon substitutes.

BRYANT: So part of building up the immune system involves depending less on drugs to do its work.

KELLERSMANN: Yes. Look at it this way. Disease is the mouse; "killer" white blood cells are the cats; antibiotics are mouse poison. If we let healthy cats do their job of eating mice, they will become more alert, more interested in their mouse-hunting, and stronger from the exercise. If we use poison to kill the mice, the cats slow down, get lazy, and may be injured themselves by the poison. So you see, the use of antibiotics is based on a dangerous principle. They can be harmful if used too often.

Of course we've learned to use that very same principle beneficially. For instance, in cases of hyperthyroidism, when a patient has a goiter—formed by the thyroid gland's overproduction of thyroxine—we introduce even more of the hormone thyroxine into the body. But in that case we want the thyroid gland to become lazy and to produce less, so that a balance is restored in the body.

BRYANT: What do antibiotics actually do in the body? How do they eliminate bacteria and disease?

KELLERSMANN: Antibiotics work either by poisoning invaders or by changing the metabolism of the invader to prevent it from multiplying.

BRYANT: Does cortisone have the same effect?

KELLERSMANN: Cortisone is actually an immune-system suppressant. It works very specifically to inhibit the workings of the lymphatic system. It has its use in cases of asthma or polioarthritis, because these are diseases in which the body's own resistance mechanism turns against itself. In such cases, we use cortisone successfully to keep the immune system from hurting the body by overreacting. But if you use cortisone on a healthy person, you're just suppressing the agents which can fight disease.

BRYANT: In most cases, then, you advocate that doctors avoid antibiotics and cortisone, and administer substances that strengthen the immune system.

KELLERSMANN: Absolutely. As far as I'm concerned, any doctor who gives antibiotics to a child or young teenager for a cold or simple infection is actually endangering his young patient's healthy development. A young person's immune system needs support so that it may develop fully. Prescribing unnecessary antibiotics is like encouraging a child to cheat in class, or like doing a young child's homework for her. Obviously, the thing is not to do the child's work for her, but to try and motivate her somehow to do her own. The problem is that this is not always the quickest, "cleanest" route.

Doctors know what they're doing, and in most cases would prefer not to use antibiotics at all. We all know that a child who takes many antibiotics will get sick again sooner than the child who has taken no antibiotics.

BRYANT: Then why do doctors do this?

KELLERSMANN: Well, of course the drug companies like it this way, and they have a great influence on medical study and practice. But even more pressure comes from the patients themselves who, in their ignorance, demand instant cures. A doctor who can't get rid of a cold in a few days is considered no good. For this reason, doctors feel forced to always take the quickest route so that they are judged to be "good doctors."

I'm very skeptical when I hear of such "good doctors," because usually that term implies that antibiotics and cortisone are used heavily in order to get rid of illnesses quickly.

BRYANT: So the "quick fix" doctor may actually be causing problems for the patient.

KELLERSMANN: Right. Because if he's using antibiotics freely, he's not strengthening the patient. Instead, he ends up actually weakening the patient's immune system.

BRYANT: Can you describe some of the biological therapies which make use of the body's natural immune system in dealing with cancer?

KELLERSMANN: I mentioned phagocytosis earlier—the process by which white blood cells actually devour the mutated cells. This natural process goes on in all of us naturally and frequently, reflecting nature's ability to cope with almost any problem on her own if given proper support.

Along these lines, one of our hopes in cancer therapy is interleukin, which stimulates the phagocytic white blood cells. Our work with interleukin—like the use of interferon or the monoclonal antibodies—has not come to a satisfactory final conclusion, but all of these processes have one thing in common: they deal with the enhancement and enforcement of the body's own immune system. This seems to be the logical direction in which to move in both cancer prevention and treatment.

BRYANT: The use of substances like interleukin seems like a rather sophisticated form of natural therapy. Somehow I've always associated European biological medicine more closely with herbs—medicinal plants.

KELLERSMANN: Yes, we use plants a great deal. For instance, we use one plant to stimulate the production of white blood cells in the body. The North American "purple cone flower," *Echinacea angustifolia* or *Echinacea purpurea* is used by most German doctors interested in natural or "biological" treatments. It's included in most cold-treatment formulas and is used for many other ailments in Europe. Native Americans used it internally and externally as well, and many American herbalists use echinacea today.

Old books dealing with naturopathic medicine discuss the plants in detail. But today, many of our medicines are manufactured from petroleum-based chemicals. Rare is the modern doctor who really knows the plants.

BRYANT: How does echinacea actually work in the body?

KELLERSMANN: Echinacea acts as a provoking agent, a nonspecific irritant to the immune system. We inject it into the veins, and the lymphatic system is stimulated to produce white blood cells in great number. This is the result we want. In the battle against cancer we need to enlist as many white-blood-cell soldiers as possible.

BRYANT: With cancer, when is it most important to stimulate the production of white blood cells?

KELLERSMANN: In cases where surgery is called for, the most critical period is right before and right after the operation. These are critical times, because during an operation there is great danger of the cancer cells being washed into other areas of the body by the bloodstream. The tumor's removal is certainly not success-ful if during the operation a bunch of cancerous cells spreads throughout the system. For this reason, it's imperative that the im-mune system be strengthened before and after surgery. However, most doctors I've spoken to don't take this precaution. Maybe they don't believe it's possible.

BRYANT: But aren't there tests which can prove that it *is* possi-ble to strengthen the immune system in this way?

KELLERSMANN: Yes. We've proven that echinacea is very effec-tive. If white blood cells are differentiated and counted in a labora-tory, and then echinacea is injected over a period of a day or two, a new white-blood-cell count will show that the number of white blood cells has increased by about twenty percent. You would think that with such proof, echinacea would be used routinely around the world.

BRYANT: Can you describe the process by which white blood cells are actually activated to deal with disease?

KELLERSMANN: White blood cells are produced and stored in the lymph nodes, in the spleen, and in the intestines. Mostly, they wait in these places like soldiers waiting in a barracks. Only a percentage act consistently as an army on its way to battle. The inactive, reserve white blood cells are called upon only when a de-structive agent appears. Then, they jump in the direction of the invader, and grab it.

BRYANT: What are some other means of fortifying one's immune system?

KELLERSMANN: We can inject the patient with thymus-gland preparations.

BRYANT: What is the function of the thymus gland?

KELLERSMANN: We are each born with a thymus gland, which sits over the heart. A baby's thymus is quite large, and gradually diminishes in size. During youth, the thymus produces hormones to protect the child by strengthening his resistance to illness. It's part of the immune system.

BRYANT: Is it true that you can heat the body up to fever-like temperatures in hopes that cancer cells will be killed at that tem-perature?

KELLERSMANN: During the process of hyperthermal thera-py, the patient is immersed in an increasingly warm tub while his pulse and body temperature are constantly measured. Heat is also applied locally; this treats the cancerous area specifically. Very simply, we're simulating a fever.

BRYANT: How does the body respond to hyperthermal therapy?

KELLERSMANN: First, many invasive agents die under the conditions of heightened temperature. Second, white blood cells immediately begin to reproduce more rapidly under feverish conditions.

It's important to realize that fever is not a disease in itself. Fever is simply the body's way of combating illness. For this reason, with an increased population of white blood cells, it's quite possible that thermal therapy might be successful against cancer, especially in early cases or after surgery, when little of the cancer remains.

BRYANT: I always considered fever to be a problem, something to fight with aspirin. I never considered that it might have therapeutic applications.

KELLERSMANN: Yes, fever is greatly misunderstood. We see it as an ailment, but the function of fever is to *fight* sickness. We should only take steps to get rid of fever when it rises to harmful levels, causing possible damage to the brain's vascular system. Even then, just cold towels should be applied; nothing more. The practice of administering medication to fight fever only serves the patient in very rare cases.

In general, a fever indicates that the body's natural healing powers are working. Fever makes the body extremely inhospitable to invading organisms. But we don't fully comprehend the mechanism that brings these higher temperatures into action. I think it's human nature, when we don't understand something, to ignore or even condemn it.

BRYANT: People of different cultures seem to have different sensitivities to the same bacteria. Is it that our immune systems have actually developed differently?

KELLERSMANN: Yes, immune systems do develop differently. The Hunza people are a good illustration of this. Historically, the Hunzas of northern Pakistan and the Himalayas have always been known to have an average life expectancy of one hundred years or more. A more vigorous, health-filled people may never be found. Yet when Western people first visited Hunza, they brought with them diseases ranging from tuberculosis to the common cold. The Hunza people actually died from the virus that produces the common cold in us.

BRYANT: If certain cultures develop immunities to particular illnesses, why can't the immune system be specifically trained to fight cancer?

KELLERSMANN: Your idea of "training" the immune system is at the root of what is called "introduced immunity." We make use of introduced immunity when we use vaccines to deal with diseases like smallpox and polio.

At birth we have no immunity to these diseases, so we build up resistance by introducing small amounts of the offending agents into the body at an early age. Of course, very small amounts of the agents are introduced — just enough for the body to recognize and react to, but not enough to make a child sick.

BRYANT: Do you envision a similar type of vaccination for cancer?

KELLERSMANN: Cancer is a different story, mainly because cancer cells inhabit our bodies normally, and our bodies fight them off without having to learn to recognize them. But it is obvious that white blood cells capable of eliminating a growing cancer are often not available in an amount large enough to cure the patient. Echinacea causes the body to produce additional white blood cells, but they're not specialized cells.

Scientists at the United States' National Cancer Institute, for instance, have worked to stimulate the cancer-fighting cells with the help of interleukin. In laboratory settings, the cancer-specific "killer cells" are produced outside the body. Once they have reproduced in large numbers, they are reinjected into the patient's bloodstream.

BRYANT: Do you think that we will one day find a prophylactic process similar to vaccination that will enable us to prevent cancer?

KELLERSMANN: Yes, I believe so. This process would surely include the administration of enzymes which fight the so-called "shielding effect." Shielding results when cholesterine (like a thin layer of fat) covers cancer cells just as it coats the walls of veins and arteries to cause arteriolosclerosis. This coating of cholesterine disguises the cells until they are unrecognizable to white blood cells programmed for phagocytosis. Enzymes help to clean these cells by removing the cholesterine.

BRYANT: Where do enzymes come from?

KELLERSMANN: The pancreas is constantly producing enzymes to be used by the intestinal system. These enzymes enter the digestive tract in the duodenum, where they mix with nourishment, break the nourishment down, and aid digestion. Anyone interested in gaining or maintaining good health must stop weakening the enzyme-producing pancreas. Enzymes are also provided through the consumption of food, especially fresh, raw vegetables and fruits.

Pancreatic enzyme production is extremely low in European and North American people because they eat so much sugar, white flour, and other processed foods. Sugar and refined foods add no enzymes to the body, and weaken the pancreas by demanding very high levels of enzyme production for digestion. The pancreas then works overtime in order to excrete the needed enzymes. A great many problems can be caused by a lack of enzymes. They have so many functions, and are so important.

BRYANT: Are there ways of supplementing the body's natural enzyme supply? Do you recommend a diet rich in high-enzyme foods?

KELLERSMANN: Yes. And in acute cases, I give my patients products prepared in Germany called Wobe-mugos and Wobe-enzymes. They are a combination of plant enzymes such as bromelain derived from pineapple, papain from papaya, and also pancreatin, the animal enzyme. Wobe-mugos can be given rectally as an enema in much higher doses than could be tolerated orally.

But more basically, to prevent cancer and other serious illness, I would suggest a healthy diet.

BRYANT: How would you describe a healthy diet?

KELLERSMANN: I use the Hunza people as an example once again, because they are reputed to have the world's highest life expectancy. First of all, they eat very little.

We, in contrast, are all used to eating far more than we need. Plus, the Hunzas eat only foods which grow in their environment; they don't import anything. They eat only *unrefined* foods: whole grains and fruits, with plenty of vitamins A and C. Water is their only drink, and their water is rich in minerals, including selenium and iron.

BRYANT: I've recently read that the blood of cancer patients is extremely low in iron.

KELLERSMANN: Yes. When iron-containing hemoglobin is at

a low level in the red blood cells, these cells find it extremely difficult to transport oxygen, especially to the cancerous area. Cancer growth may indicate a condition of low oxygen.

Oxygen helps to metabolize our nourishment properly. Without enough oxygen, we can't make efficient use of the foods we eat; without oxygen, our fuel cannot be burned.

First, nutrients are broken down with the help of enzymes. Then red blood cells do the rest to supply every part of the body with the oxygen it needs to function properly.

BRYANT: What exactly is the role of the red blood cell?

KELLERSMANN: The red blood cell's role is to supply the body with oxygen. The more hemoglobin the red blood cells have, the greater the cells' capacity to carry oxygen.

BRYANT: Are there foods which can actually help the body to increase its oxygen supply?

KELLERSMANN: Yes. Dr. Seeger from East Germany has found that plants and juices like red grapes and beets—foods containing a lot of red color—seem to increase the percentage of oxygen in the body. Allegedly, they contain agents which supplement the oxygen-carrying capacities of red blood cells.

BRYANT: Basically, you seem to think that eating whole foods and living simply, close to nature, is the best way to guard one's health.

KELLERSMANN: Yes. Nature has found the best way of keeping us alive. We should not be so bold as to think that we can improve upon mother nature's plan. First we must cut down on those "civilized," refined foods. We must stop eating breakfasts of white toast, jam and coffee. That's no breakfast —that's garbage! Jam, for instance, is sugar—little more than refined sugar. Sugar robs us of so many B-vitamins that we're weakened before we walk out the door. The loss of B-vitamins lowers our resistance to stress and contributes to frequent sickness.

It's ironic that many nutritionists still insist that sugar is "pure" energy. They never mention the energy which is drained from the body in order to react to this "pure" energy.

Refined sugar is a shock to the nervous system, which may be one reason we civilized people are always running around like maniacs. We eat too much sugar, sometimes without even knowing that it's included in the foods we're eating. Our bodies are then involved in the process of coping with it. The reality is that sugar weakens us tremendously.

BRYANT: Does coffee have a similar effect?

KELLERSMANN: Coffee, like sugar, jacks up the nervous system so quickly that the body is pushed out of balance. Also, both coffee and sugar overstimulate the adrenal glands and the nerves, which must compensate. This is why we have that very low feeling when sugar or caffeine wears off. True to the old maxim, the higher you climb, the deeper you fall.

BRYANT: Does constant manipulation of the adrenal and nervous systems make the body more prone to attack by cancerous or other mutant cells?

KELLERSMANN: Physical abuse of any kind, including dietary abuse, weakens our bodies' ability to fight disease. It's as simple as that. The whole problem today is that we're always in a hurry. That's why doctors feel they must cure us in one day. That's why when we feel low, we eat candy bars which give a quick lift, but then drain us, instead of apples, which would add helpful digestive enzymes. We are always pushing ourselves, and we push the pancreas to work harder and harder by eating refined foods, which have been separated from the biological complex designed for wholesome nourishment.

BRYANT: Obviously then, parents should avoid giving candy to their children.

KELLERSMANN: Giving candy to children is harmful. Why not give children fruits, seeds and nuts? We're simply too involved with the habit of eating candy and other junk foods which claim to offer our bodies "instant energy." The wrappers never tell us of the strain produced in the body by such foods. They never mention the letdown that follows.

BRYANT: In the U.S., where the Food and Drug Administration puts a warning on each cigarette package, maybe there should also be warning labels on candy bars.

KELLERSMANN: Yes, saying, "If you don't want to be damaged by eating this instant-energy product, you should take a B-vitamin supplement and then lie down."

But then you have children eating French fries and soda for lunch, which may even be worse than candy. With this lunch, children are eating the burned, saturated fat in which the potatoes have been cooked. This fat, producing benzopyric nitrates, becomes carcinogenic when it begins to smoke, as its chemical composition changes with the heat. Then there are the potatoes, which

have been skinned of their vitamins and have very little nutritional value. Salt is put on top of them, which is hard on the kidneys.
Finally, the soda: just water and sugar. What a lunch for a child!
But it happens all the time. Kids nowadays want nothing else. Their
mothers say, "What shall we give them to eat? They want only this
junk food. They'll eat nothing else." Well, eating nothing might actually be better than eating the foods I've just described. We can
only be as healthy as the food we give ourselves. Maybe this sounds
simplistic to many people, but good health really can be such a
simple thing.

Nutrition should be every nation's priority, and we should be
electing people who think more about the safety and health of the
people. How can our nations be strong if our people are not?

BRYANT: Do you ever advise your cancer patients to change their
lifestyles or at least their diets?

KELLERSMANN: For people with relatively healthy habits, survival may be enhanced by continuing to live normally. That's because a great deal of stress is associated with change of any kind.
But someone who is constantly under pressure, eats white toast
with jam for breakfast every morning, and generally lives an unhealthy life, should make changes.

When it's a matter of life and death, people find the strength
to change. Some choose to continue with business as usual. In
general, relaxed yet active people have greater chances of staying
healthy than people who are under constant stress or people who
are completely unfamiliar with good dietary habits.

BRYANT: Is there an age or a period of life during which cancer
is most dangerous?

KELLERSMANN: Since cancer cells are body cells, they multiply and grow as quickly as the body itself grows. Children tend
to have what I call dangerous "racing-car" cancers, which reproduce and grow quite quickly. Older people have "bicycle speed"
cancers. Growth is slow, and so for elderly people, conventional
cancer treatment such as chemotherapy, x-ray and surgery may very
well do more harm than good.

BRYANT: Many people are interested in learning about cancer
detection. What diagnostic methods do you use?

KELLERSMANN: Personally, I use chemical tests including
blood analyses, which measure concentrations of trace minerals,
hemoglobin, white blood cells, and immune system indicators such
as carcinomic embryonic antibodies—the body's response to can-

cer. I administer blood tests routinely. I look for low iron and high copper content in the blood, and many other factors.

In general, I believe that mastery of diagnosis is based not on a narrow focus, but on the diagnostician's own thoughtfulness and breadth of vision.

So I use all kinds of methods. I examine my patients' eyes for changes in the irises. I observe my patients' closely. I listen to them. I try not to jump to conclusions. When someone says, "Drinking coffee makes me feel awful," I don't immediately say, "That's gall-bladder." I wait until I have lots of other evidence to support that idea. I try to keep an open mind until a combination of signals, gained from a variety of diagnostic methods, points to one thing rather narrowly. Then I confirm or dispute my hypothesis with a blood test, and other tests. I never rely on one test or one diagnosis.

BRYANT: Can you describe your own method of cancer treatment?

KELLERSMANN: In the case of a tumorous cancer, I make use of surgery because it allows us to remove a tremendous burden from the body. After the operation, I might use radiation to kill the cells surrounding the tumor.

BRYANT: In general then, you follow a conventional protocol.

KELLERSMANN: Except for the fact that I give enzymes before and after the operation. Wobe-mugos and Wobe-enzymes can be taken in high concentrations. Second, I give thymus injections after the operation. Third, I strengthen the body's own resistance by increasing the number of white blood cells through echinacea injections, and through high doses of vitamin A.

Nutritionally speaking, I give the patient only food which allows the pancreas to work normally—no junk food. This allows for efficient enzyme use by the pancreas, and keeps the nervous and adrenaline systems from being jacked up and down. I also make sure that the intestines are cleaned out daily by giving bulky foods.

BRYANT: You've mentioned that oxygen is especially important to the cancer patient.

KELLERSMANN: Yes. And as many oncologists have suggested, the oxygen available to the body can be increased by diet. Of course, oxygen should also be present in the form of a healthy environment of good, clean air. Cancer patients should be exposed to lots of oxygen after their operations. In short, I try to treat my cancer patients with an awareness of how both physical and psychological factors affect and contribute to a patient's well-being.

My position is that the natural, biological treatments I've mentioned are neither the best treatments nor the only treatments.
I strongly urge that we combine treatments. There is no reason
not to have the best of both worlds. We should complement modern technology with our knowledge of nutrition, natural immunity, and other basic aspects of human life and health.

BRYANT: What is the most important part of your cancer-
treatment program?

KELLERSMANN: Strengthening the immune system! Every
doctor knows that the body's own white blood cells are normally
capable of doing away with cancerous cells. So if we want to prevent cancer or fight cancer, particularly the cancer which may
spread after an operation, we must increase the number of white
blood cells.   The wisdom of nature, like all wisdom, is that which
is simplest. In cancer treatment, this means that the immune system should be a primary consideration in the treatment of cancer. Only now, in response to the AIDS crisis and growing incidents
of cancer, is the immune system taken seriously by science as an
element of possible treatment.

We should be broadening our approach to include more than
just the two or three methods produced by the chemical indus-
tries. We have to recognize that we're natural, living beings. We
can cooperate with nature instead of trying to ignore her.

We've become so egotistical that we'll only accept those things
we've invented ourselves. We've invented chemotherapy, but as you
know, we haven't invented our natural system of immunity. So we
ignore its function and its importance.

BRYANT: What you're describing sounds like a kind of arrogance.

KELLERSMANN: Yes, but as they say, pride comes before a fall.
Overconfidence leads us to change and cover up what exists, instead of adapting to those conditions. We don't want the heat; we
don't want the cold; we don't want the insects; we don't want to
age. We want to change it all—to reinvent it all. We think we can
improve on everything. It seems that we've lost our humility before nature. We've forgotten that we're a part of her. We laugh at
prayer, joking that God is a nagging old man with a long, white
beard. We forget to be humble in facing the natural forces which
are greater than ourselves. Instead, we want to ignore all the forces
which we can't influence.

BRYANT: Doesn't this attitude reach far beyond cancer
treatment?

KELLERSMANN: Yes, especially as the frontier of modern science gets involved with practices like gene manipulation and cloning. If we don't learn to treat and prevent cancer and other health problems in nature's own way, we may, through our own pride, fail to save human beings from destruction on a greater level.

The Planet is our Body

T'AI SITUPA

An adept of Tibetan medicine, Lama T'ai Situpa is an accomplished master of meditation and one of the foremost leaders and teachers of Tibetan Buddhism's Kagyupa lineage. As an expression of his commitment to help bring about world peace, he is founder and director of Maitreya Institute, a multicultural educational organization offering classes, workshops, seminars, performances, and ongoing exchange among diverse disciplines in the arts and sciences.

When still a child in 1959, T'ai Situpa escaped from Chinese-occupied Tibet along with thousands of other Tibetans. As part of the Indo-Tibetan tradition of transferring knowledge and power from one generation to another, he and other young regents of Kagyu Buddhism were raised and personally schooled by the Gyalwa Karmapa at the Rhumtek Monastery in Gantok, Sikkim. Today, T'ai Situpa is recognized as a great lama who, with his understanding of Western culture, successfully communicates Buddhist teachings in English. Much of the information described herein reflects T'ai Situpa's study of the classic Tibetan scholarly works, including the principal medical text Gyu-zhi. This text from the eighth century reflects traditional knowledge and wisdom of Indian, Chinese, Persian, Greek, and Tibetan cultures.

51

INTRODUCTION

After working on this book for two years, I reviewed my progress with T'ai Situpa. At the time, my work reflected a polarization of opinions and approaches within the medical community. T'ai Situpa responded to me by pointing out that I must see everyone's perspective and contribution to the process of working with cancer not as right or wrong, but simply as "part of the evolution." This helped me to see that there was no need to take sides or judge those with different orientations. At that point, I began to ask questions more objectively, with a more open mind. Instead of writing a book on the one true "cure" for cancer, I became more committed to showing a number of different, complementary viewpoints. My goal became to provide a useful forum for intercultural dialogue which would benefit both individuals searching for personal answers and society at large.

The Indo-Tibetan perspective and system of logic are as evolved as our own, but differ from ours in many ways. Interconnectedness, interdependence and all-inclusiveness characterize the Tibetan way, which is concerned with cause and effect and the relationship between life on Earth and the planet itself.

As a result, T'ai Situpa helped me to become more aware of our human responsibility to speak up about our vital relationship with the Earth and with all forms of life. And in relation to cancer and the process of healing, T'ai Situpa has inspired me to think in ways that go beyond the limits of my own education and cultural limitations.

DIALOGUE

T'AI SITUPA: Although our human bodies are quite small, we have many big ideas about ourselves. These ideas and preconceptions make it very hard for us to understand some of the problems we face today. Our planet, however, is more like an object to us; we don't have as many ideas about the Earth as we do about our own bodies.

We should always remember that our presence here on this Earth is absolutely essential to our humanness. Thanks to the Earth we are physical beings. Our relationship with the planet is the very thing that allows us to experience life not just on the mental or spiritual level, but also on the physical level.

Since we and the Earth are so closely related, and since it is easier to calmly observe a planet than it is to calmly observe our own selves, the planet may offer us many important opportunities to learn about ourselves.

BRYANT: Are you suggesting that we consider the Earth to be a reflection of our own bodies, somehow?

T'AI SITUPA: Not a reflection, exactly. According to the principles of Tibetan medicine, the planet *is* our body. Our body is the planet. We share characteristics with the planet; thus, it is possible to live on this Earth. If you read Tibetan texts such as the *Abhidharma* or the *Gyu-zhi*, you can glimpse the traditional Tibetan perspective on relationships between the human body and the body of our planet. These texts explain that we're part of this planet, and that people and even the Earth itself enjoy health or have illnesses, partly as a result of this close relationship.

BRYANT: Would you say then that we actually share diseases with the Earth? Cancer, for instance?

T'AI SITUPA: If we observe the planet carefully, we see evidence that the Earth itself is being affected by the things that affect us. We might even say that the surface of our planet is being invaded by cancerous activity. Learning about how this might have happened to the Earth, we may learn a great deal about the human body. Discovering ways to remedy the situation on Earth will surely parallel the discovery of ways to cure ourselves. And these ways will be in harmony with the Earth.

BRYANT: What is your perspective on the recent widespread appearance of life-threatening diseases such as cancer or AIDS?

T'AI SITUPA: Today we have a lot of unfamiliar diseases, which are difficult to deal with scientifically. They become "dread diseases" when our bodies are unable to cope with them.

BRYANT: Why do you think this is this occurring now?

T'AI SITUPA: One very obvious reason is that since 1945 we have experienced more than five hundred nuclear explosions on our planet, in the name of research and for reasons of aggression. These explosions are still affecting the atmosphere of the entire planet tremendously; thus they affect our bodies tremendously as well.

Nuclear waste is another problem. We know that this waste is poison, and we know that it will not disappear by itself. It leaks into our atmosphere and into the earth itself, and we don't know how to take care of it.

Also, people today are using all kinds of chemicals. Many are almost addicted or dependent upon these chemicals, which range from perfumes, deodorants and food preservatives to purifying chemicals added to our water. These chemicals are very powerful, and they too have a great effect on people.

BRYANT: In the evolution of life on Earth, these are relatively new products, phenomena which human bodies haven't had to deal with before, especially in such large amounts.

T'AI SITUPA: Right. Although the individual chemical substances making up these products have existed, these new compounds had never been made. Our ancestors never knew these substances, which are actually very hard for us to get adjusted to in the short time allowed us: a generation, or even just a few years.

BRYANT: Many people are concerned about our overconsumption of refined foods for that very reason.

T'AI SITUPA: Food is the biggest single factor affecting everybody's health. Before, food came direct from the planet. Once, we didn't use pesticides to kill other natural beings. If there were insects or something in the crops, people would do some spiritual practice—use some gentle way of cleansing the environment.

For example, in Tibet, when a big field is eaten up by rats, the lamas offer the Rat Blessing. It is a complex prayer, but the message is basically, "All the rats of this area, you should not eat what is growing here on this farm." Then the rats simply do not eat from the farm. Under the right conditions, I would say that the same thing can be done for bacteria and for everything else.

BRYANT: The Rat Blessing is so very far away from the kind of farming techniques practiced by Westerners.

T'AI SITUPA: That's because life is so different here. In Tibet you know everyone who lives around you for twenty miles in every direction. Here in America the people who live in apartment houses may not even know who lives above or below them or even next door. If people don't have the time or aren't interested in communicating with each other, how will they communicate with the animals, plants or other forms of life? Maybe they don't. But it's really a very natural thing to be doing.

It's interesting to me that scientists are now trying to replicate the structure of plants, chemically, in the laboratory. But it would take many years to make even one chemical with the power of an entire plant—even the smallest of plants. And in the end, would it really be the same? Why not just go to the mountain, pick the plant, and learn to understand the plant? It's there. It's natural. You don't have to take years and millions of dollars. You don't have to make lots of mistakes. The plant is just perfect the way it is, reflecting the health or the weakness of the earth itself.

We're connected with our atmosphere and our Earth in many ways. Concrete, practical examples of how we're connected with the planet are discussed in the ancient Tibetan texts, which also describe which herbs to use as medicine, even when and where to pick them and how they should be prepared. It's ancient knowledge that our ancestors have known for hundreds of years.

BRYANT: Would you say that herbs are especially effective because they share the qualities of the Earth with us?

T'AI SITUPA: All medicine shares the qualities of the Earth. Even the modern medicines which we call "chemicals" are derived from substances found naturally on this planet. The difference is that some forms of life are perfect for us to use just as they're found in nature; they're food and medicine in one. Tibetan medical science tells us how these products can be used to balance the body without harming it—without causing side effects. For this reason, I believe, the plants themselves are especially valuable.

BRYANT: What are your thoughts on the path of scientific and technological progress that we, the people of the twentieth century, have chosen to follow?

T'AI SITUPA: There are two kinds of evolution: slow and steady, and fast and shaky. We're experiencing a very shaky, fast evolution. What's happened to us within this past hundred years has happened much faster and much more dramatically than what happened to our ancestors during the thousand or ten thousand years before. Today, everything changes quickly. Because it changes so fast, people get into so many things; the confusion surrounding people is very obvious. It's almost as if we were constantly jumping from a pool of ice into a pool of nearly boiling water. You jump into hot water and almost get cooked, and then jump back into cold water and almost get frozen. Then after you jump once more back into the hot water and almost get cooked, it's time to jump back into the cold pool and freeze. Just like that. It's sudden shock.

BRYANT: What can we do about this, other than slow down?

T'AI SITUPA: I'm not actually sure that it's necessary or even possible to slow down. But *we do have to relax.* We have to relax so that we can understand this age. Then we'll see the best way to deal with it. If we're able to relax and relate to a situation properly, there's nothing that can't be worked out. With a relaxed mind, there is no madness.

BRYANT: What do you think has caused all this accelerated tension and rush?

T'AI SITUPA: I don't like to think that it's somebody's fault. It's simply happening. The rush is simply a part of our evolution. That's all.

BRYANT: I think that the pace we keep has something to do with the fact that, in this century, we're so involved with machines that we tend to see our own bodies as machines. We lose sight of the fragile balance and precious nature of human existence.

T'AI SITUPA: Certainly, we must come to appreciate the value and importance of the human body, all living bodies, the Earth body, all of life. This will definitely happen, although right now it seems we can't even begin to catch up. We have little time for reflection, so we get confused. It's as if the faster things go, the longer it takes. It will take some time.

BRYANT: Do you think that our major health problems, including increased cancer incidence, are somehow related to this speeding-up process?

T'AI SITUPA: It may be. Just think of the food we eat. You can eat Chinese food in America and American food in China. You can eat Middle Eastern food in Europe, and European food in the Middle East. Or you can fly from Hawaii to Beijing for a lunch in China. Then off to the Middle East for Arabic food. Later on you can go straight to London for English food. So within twenty-four hours you can experience three different atmospheres and three different diets. People take this for granted and think there's nothing strange about it, but I don't think it's normal. You really give your physical condition a hard time if you're constantly making it adjust to a new environment every few hours.

Every place yields its food, which is perfect for that set of physical conditions. The food of each place has been feeding generations of people for centuries. There is always a strong connection between the food of a region and the people living in that region.

BRYANT: Our ancestors worked the same land for generations, and the food they ate often came either from their own land or from a neighbor's.

T'AI SITUPA: Yes, and in those days, it would take a whole day to go even twenty miles. Let's say a trip from California to Alaska was made on foot or on horseback. Every day, gradually, the travelers would acclimate themselves to the climatic changes and different food available. That's the natural way. Today, things are going too fast in too short a time. Just jumping back and forth the way we do, our whole system gets confused. We don't realize how these things affect us, but everything does have an effect. That's why so many unusual things happen to us. That's why we have so many social problems, including the diseases you've mentioned. It's not a matter of stopping our travels. But we should be aware that everything we do has an effect on us. Awareness of the effects of our actions can prevent many problems.

BRYANT: Do you think we might find an antidote to all this?

T'AI SITUPA: Prevention is better than an antidote. The important thing to do is to relax while being cautious. We need to relate to our conditions in appropriate ways, from a relaxed point of view. It may be that the cause and cure of cancer is something rather simple—something that we're overlooking—an idea that's simply unfamiliar to us in this modern culture.

The important thing to remember is that everything really is connected. We all breathe the same air along with the insects, germs and plants. And when the properties of our atmosphere change, we're all affected. To give an example, humans insist upon cutting and re-shaping the Earth without thinking, in order to make tunnels and highways. This changes the energy of the Earth, but we don't notice the changes. Human beings often act in ignorance, and in this way we do a great deal of damage.

Of course it's also important to remember that not all imbalances are caused by humans. Volcanoes, earthquakes and other activities take their own natural course. The Earth's way of correcting itself may not be consistent with the human being's idea of how things should be. But in the end, there will be balance.

BRYANT: The idea of a self-correcting, balancing force in nature offers a great deal of hope.

T'AI SITUPA: Yes, and we can all remember that we're also part of that balancing force. We're involved in it. It's not just something happening outside of us.

BRYANT: Lama Kalu Rinpoche once talked about future imbalances on this planet. He mentioned that in the future the human life span will be reduced. How does his prediction fit in with some of the things you've presented here?

T'AI SITUPA: According to the Buddhist scriptures, human life will become shorter both in length and also in value. The value of life will change drastically. The meaningful work you can do now within ten years may take one whole lifetime to do in the future. This doesn't mean that people will not be busy; they'll be busier than ever. But when they die they will have accomplished less. A few thousand years back, people learned a lot in one lifetime. Many could attain enlightenment in one lifetime. Now only a few can do that, because of the pace of life today. So much to do, and so little getting done.

BRYANT: Is there a practical solution?

T'AI SITUPA: We have so many bombs and so much waste. We use so many cars and so much fuel. Production has gone beyond the point of being useful. In fact, it's quite chaotic—out of control. Why not find ways of traveling which make use of gravity or solar energy instead of fossil fuel? Surely that would be more effective, more economical and more healing.

The solution will come when we can all participate in practical ways. The solution will involve all of us doing the things that are truly necessary. It means that we must stop doing and making unnecessary things. That's one solution.

BRYANT: Can you talk about a cure for cancer, specifically?

T'AI SITUPA: On one level, the Tibetans have developed a special medicine from detoxified mercury. I have complete faith in it.

It's interesting to note that cancer itself, like quicksilver, has many different natures. In Tibetan medicine, we have specific medicines for every specific nature of a disease. Cancer may develop in the lungs, the stomach, the liver, the blood. Thus, specific medicines are administered along with the refined quicksilver to treat the part or parts of the body affected by the cancer. The refined quicksilver takes the medicine to the point in the body where it is needed. It's very powerful. It goes where there's a problem — nowhere else. It's a vehicle for the medicine.

But I've also described another kind of cure for cancer: to stop making what we don't need, to stop creating so much waste. This could be seen as a type of ultimate cure.

BRYANT: We've been led to believe that our planet is an inanimate object. This attitude contributes to a lack of respect for our environment. What is the Tibetan Buddhist view of the actual nature of the Earth?

T'AI SITUPA: You could ask, "Between the human body and the Earth body, which is more animate?" The answer is that they are both exactly the same. The human body is no more animate than the Earth. Mind inhabits the human body, but the human body is simply the host. When a person dies, the body is still there — like a dead tree. It decomposes.

BRYANT: But the live human body has a consciousness. Does the planet Earth have a consciousness?

T'AI SITUPA: That's hard to say, but by Buddhist principles, why not? This planet may represent just the tiniest drop of sweat of another sentient being. In that sense, it may very well be animate, just as your finger or your toe is animate. You can say that you're a part of the Earth and that the entire Earth is part of you because you're here and you're connected to the Earth. So does the Earth share in that consciousness? Is the Earth itself conscious? You could certainly say so.

BRYANT: So all the billions of conscious beings populating the Earth could simply be a part of a much greater, collective consciousness?

T'AI SITUPA: Interdependent beings performing interdependent actions. Yes.

BRYANT: With the political situation of the world the way it is, it's hard to recognize even human interdependence sometimes. We divide ourselves so easily into opposing teams. Yet faced with disease and other threats to the existence of life as we know it, it seems more and more important to meet the challenge of living in harmony with our environment.

Our efforts to live in harmony may bring even "enemies" like capitalist and communist powers toward increased cooperation. What do you see as a good starting point for this sort of activity? What will it take for the leaders of the world to go beyond their own belief systems and self-interest, to find a solution for the global problems we face?

T'AI SITUPA: I think that everyone has to relax and put aside personal interests. I think that our political leaders have to ask themselves why they're leading their countries. What is the purpose? What is motivating them? They must have clear, relaxed sincerity in what they're doing. If people's goals and motivations are toward good ends, things will begin to change and go in that direction. If their motivation is bad, then the outcome of their actions will go in that very same direction.

Certainly, if people are involved in deciding the best method of killing one another, they will not be benefiting anyone. They just have to see and know that.

BRYANT: It's difficult for the leaders of large countries to get the kind of perspective that would enable them to focus their attention on the greater common good. They're embroiled in crises which seem to demand instant and profitable solutions. And they're all limited by the needs and demands of their own constituencies.

T'AI SITUPA: We really should take all the presidents and foreign ministers to another planet so that they can gain some perspective and see their stupidity: a big hammer in the right hand, a big knife in the left hand. This is to bash this one; that is to chop that one. We're like that. We're so small down here on this insignificant little planet, and yet we fight among ourselves over territory—over everything.

But the planet is not our property. It belongs to the fish; it belongs to the birds; it belongs to the deer; it belongs to the trees; it also belongs to people. But it's not our exclusive property.

BRYANT: In this age, we're dealing with many challenging situations that may, in all their difficulty, actually help us to progress toward becoming a united planet. Specifically now, I'm thinking about cancer and AIDS. Can you talk about how people might use such individual hardship on the path of personal growth or liberation?

T'AI SITUPA: Cancer and AIDS are as good as anything on the path of liberation. Any disease or any difficulty may play the same role. It's not just these two. One can learn and benefit from absolutely anything. You might have a difficult wife or husband, or terrible kids. Then you can really learn lessons, such as how to be patient. You can learn a great deal from any difficult situation.

BRYANT: By making that situation an ally instead of an enemy?

T'AI SITUPA: Yes. One way of using disease as an ally would be to decide on a treatment you want to follow, follow that treatment, and get well. In the case of cancer, perhaps you decide to dedicate yourself to cancer research. You could also dedicate all the suffering of having the disease to the benefit of others.

In Tibet, where people are conscious of having chosen the conditions of each lifetime or incarnation, the work of healing involves physical exercises which are also spiritually beneficial. These exercises may involve going around holy Mount Kailash on foot, for instance, and maybe doing prostrations all around the mountain. Or water might be collected from a special, holy area and drunk. Other people get well doing spiritual exercises while taking special medicines. Still others don't even take the medicine. They just do the spiritual practice and get well. Many Tibetan people meditate on the image of the Medicine Buddha, source of all healing.

The important thing to remember is that everything begins in the mind. Mind is the most important thing. If one is relaxed, if one can accept what is, then the medicine power — the power of any treatment — is much more effective. Here in America there are nonreligious ways of healing by working with both the mental and physical together: music therapy, exercise therapy, special diet. The idea is to calm the mind and encourage positive thinking.

BRYANT: Can you talk more about the Medicine Buddha — what he represents and some of his special qualities?

T'AI SITUPA: Medicine Buddha is the healing aspect of the Buddha. That's the way Buddha manifested when he taught medicine here on Earth. The essential qualities of the Medicine Buddha are enlightened compassion, loving kindness and wisdom. We say that the essence of the Medicine Buddha is Dharmakaya — all-pervading truth.

BRYANT: How would you suggest that people visualize or tap into the essence of the Medicine Buddha? Not just practitioners of Buddhism, but anyone who would like to develop the healing qualities within.

T'AI SITUPA: Communicating with one's disease is a good and correct way. This may involve learning about the illness and then accepting a means of dealing with it, such as eating the right foods, taking the correct medication, living in a way that helps to heal the sickness, while trying to understand the connections between your body, your mind, the planet, and even the atmosphere surrounding you.

In terms of future generations, we really must improve the way we educate people, the way we modify people's attitudes and the way we provide them with skills. If we're not successful in educating our people, we end up having to discipline them — restraining them or locking them up.

I also think we have to somehow eliminate our habits of weakness: weak thinking habits, talking and listening habits, eating habits, living habits. We have to make improvements so that we can enjoy rich, high-quality lives — so that we can utilize our lives properly. Then we'll be doing well.

BRYANT: Many people, including cancer patients, have begun to use visualization as a means of learning and healing. Can you recommend any visualization techniques that would be helpful for people to practice?

T'AI SITUPA: This is an individual matter. There are many types of visualization. But even more effective is the actual day-to-day practice of loving kindness. The practice of loving kindness is the secular healing practice. It is open to everyone, and it really is the most effective, universal way.

BRYANT: What is the most important message you would like to share about disease and the process of healing?

T'AI SITUPA: The most important things are really very simple. First, we must all take very good care of our health; we must know the value of health. At the same time we have to take good care of our minds. We shouldn't choose chaotic activities. We should be more aware of what we're doing — not only in terms of our physical actions, but also in terms of our intentions and motivations.

We have to be aware and mindful. We have to be as relaxed and calm as possible. Then, most importantly, we have to have "good heart." Kindness is the universal religion. Acceptance of other ways of thinking and being is a part of that kindness.

The Concerns of a Radiologist

SEYMOUR BRENNER, M.D.

Dr. Seymour Brenner is a therapeutic radiologist with a private practice in Brooklyn, New York. Since 1951 he has served on two chapters of the American Cancer Society, and is active as a member of Brooklyn's radiology review board. He served as attending physician in radiology at Maimonides Medical Center for twenty years, and is currently director of radiotherapy at Peninsula General Hospital in Far Rockaway, New York.

A diplomate of the American Board of Radiology, Dr. Brenner is a member of the Kings County New York Medical Society, the American College of Radiology, the Brooklyn Radiological Society, the New York Radiological Society, and the American Society of Therapeutic Radiologists. His written contributions to the field have been published in Clinical Research, *the* New York Journal of Medicine, Cancer Chemotherapy Reports, Cancer, *and other journals.*

INTRODUCTION

During our first meeting, Dr. Brenner expressed a love of helping others as well as a great eagerness to communicate his knowledge. His willingness to candidly share his own experiences, gleaned from thirty-five years of work in the cancer field, contributed to many subsequent dialogues. In the process, however, he also communicated a tremendous sense of frustration due to lack of progress in his field, high patient mortality, and other obstacles to attaining personal fulfillment through his work. During the months and years that have followed, I've found that this syndrome of frustration is very common among conscientious physicians.

I sat in Dr. Brenner's waiting room more than thirty times over the course of one year, accompanying a friend with cancer. This experience offered me many opportunities to appreciate how precious the human body is, how easy it is to lose.

In the reception room, I'm conscious that each waiting person could be the subject of an entire book. I feel the anxiety in each pair of eyes, the concern in the face of each loved one accompanying a patient. The office attendants are always efficient, and show concern and kindness for each patient. But I feel an atmosphere of guarded caution. Medical history forms are filled out. Suspense is in the air. Optimism is tempered by fear. Is there a word for "conditional hope?"

While patients prepare for treatment, circles made with medical magic marker designate targets for radiation on the skin of children, old people, middle-aged men and women wearing hospital gowns buttoned up the back. So much preparation for just thirty seconds of treatment is disorienting. Yet Dr. Brenner's concern offers an almost palpable sense of support.

I greatly appreciated these opportunities to gain insight into the workings of a radiotherapist's office, but my contact with cancer patients there made me aware that I was living in a privileged observer's world. Upon leaving I could cherish my relatively good health.

Marveling at the extent of human knowledge, I understood that radiotherapy is the fruit of our ability to harness a tremendous natural power in order to heal. At the same time, I was aware that radiation can cause cancer as well as cure it. It seemed painfully ironic that while advances in technology have contributed to so much cancer through radiation, our solution is to then have our cells irradiated as a cure.

Dialogue with Dr. Brenner encouraged my interest in the field of oncology. His patience and openness allowed me to feel comfortable as a lay person asking basic medical questions; and his willingness to share information, thoughts and feelings as both doctor and friend has distinguished him among patients as well as among other members of the medical community on a national level.

DIALOGUE

A PRIVATE PRACTICE IN RADIOLOGY

BRYANT: Could you describe the actual work that you do? What is radiation, exactly, and how does it work, especially as a form of cancer therapy?

BRENNER: Radiation is a form of energy which has the specific quality of penetrability. Although it may be produced by certain elements such as radium and cobalt, we generally use radiation produced by electricity.

When you turn on an ordinary electric light bulb, the filament produces electrons. Likewise, when you turn on the light bulb in an x-ray tube, the filament lights up and produces electrons. These electrons are then drawn by an electrical field across space until they hit a target. Upon hitting that target, x-rays are produced. Voltage determines the rate at which those electrons move through space; the rate of the electrons' travel determines the penetrability of the beam that's produced.

The penetrability of an x-ray made with one million volts of electricity is much greater than the penetrability of a one-hundred volt x-ray. We normally use between one to eight million volts of electricity in cancer treatment, because high levels of energy radiation are needed to penetrate tissues deep in the body.

BRYANT: I've often heard the word "rads" referring to radiation dosage. How do rads relate to voltage?

BRENNER: Rads are units of radiation dosage which measure the amount of energy deposited per gram of tissue. Electron volts actually control the flow of radiation and thus the dosage itself, measured in rads.

BRYANT: How does the penetration of radiation into body tissue act therapeutically?

BRENNER: In treating cancer, radiation alters a cell's metabolic potential. It destroys the cell's ability to anabolize — to build. Primarily, radiation affects the division of cells. When cells have been irradiated, very often they can't divide. Even if the irradiated cells do divide, their ability to reproduce is most often impaired, and so they die out.

Another point is that cells from different areas of the body have different characteristics. If you look under a microscope at a kidney cell, you'll see it differs greatly from a lung cell. But the theory behind radiation is that all cells which have become malignant, be they kidney cells, lung cells, brain cells or whatever, metabolize more rapidly than normal cells, and their reproductive cycles are shorter. Therefore, a normal cell which is irradiated may live for thirty days after being irradiated, whereas an irradiated cancer cell may only live for two days.

Because of their rapid division and short reproductive cycle, cancer cells are theoretically more sensitive to the alteration of their metabolism by radiation than are normal cells.

BRYANT: Dealing with radiation as therapy, you treat cancer patients exclusively. Is that right?

BRENNER: Yes, all of my patients are cancer patients with proven malignancies. Before coming here, the typical patient has already run the gamut in searching for medical care. First, he or she has gone to a family practitioner or internist who originally suspected a malignancy, then to a surgeon, who most likely established the diagnosis. The surgeon may decide to send the patient to a chemotherapist. The chemotherapist may subsequently decide that the patient should be seen by me as a radiotherapist.

Each of my patients has been referred to me after a diagnosis has been made by another physician who feels that I can help. Each patient comes here with a disease which has already been diagnosed as cancer. Now, it's up to me to decide whether radiotherapy has a promising role in treatment. If I decide that it does, I discuss that with the patient and with the patient's family. We talk over what I intend to do and what the outlook is, because I believe that patients should know.

I then administer a course of treatment from beginning to end, and finally I refer the patient back to his or her physician, usually to the internist or family practitioner who maintains day-to-day care. The care of cancer patients is not one doctor's work; it is the work of the several physicians who may be involved with patients' treatment.

BRYANT: In observing your practice, I see that though you treat up to forty patients a day, you have some special gifts which allow you to work with each of them each in a warm and caring way. Can you talk about your approach to your patients and to medicine in general?

BRENNER: To begin with, although I'm a radiologist, my work involves more than just administering radiation. I also use a personal system of support and counsel that I've developed through the years of working with people in my role as physician.

First I discuss with each patient his or her particular condition and outlook. Then we talk about what we are going to do. And to be perfectly frank, most patients are literally scared out of their wits—terrified, and justifiably so—faced with issues of life and death of their own.

So my speech to every patient deals with facing up to the fact that each of us will die, and with the idea that the trick in life is to live *well* until we die. If cancer patients live in fear, then they will be depriving themselves of the very joy in life that they're fearful of losing through death. So we establish first that death is inevitable, that no one knows whose day is next, and that your having cancer doesn't mean that you'll die before me. It can happen to any one of us at any time. Worrying about it is self-defeating.

I always give them an example of my own problems. For instance, while they're fearful of dying of cancer, I happen to be living with a threat of blindness. So I tell them, "I know that I'll probably go blind before I die. But should the fact that I'm going to go blind five years from now cause me to stop seeing today? No. If you have cancer, you shouldn't stop living today just because you're afraid you might die tomorrow."

BRYANT: Can you talk about some of the emotions that you and your patients have to deal with?

BRENNER: I have seen anger and a great deal of fear, but very often those emotions come not from the patient as much as from his next of kin. Healthy relatives will come in here and say to me in privacy, "Can't you put my husband or my wife in some institution? I can't be bothered with it." I think this comes from fear—fear, when you see a loved one dying, that your own turn is not far away. So these people are angry that their relatives with cancer are reminding them of death.

In this office, though, more than anger or outright fear, I have seen depression. Depression and frustration are the conditions I have to deal with most.

BRYANT: Most of us want to believe that our bodies are like machines, invulnerable and immortal.

BRENNER: Well, people learn very quickly when they sit down here that it's simply not so. We are all going to die. My patients are confronted with the fact that death is inevitable for all of us.

I'm not saying that cancer is not a threatening disease. Having cancer may mean that your life is more acutely threatened than the life of someone else. However, my treatment may keep you alive long enough to outlive your mate and lots of other people you know. The one thing I can actually guarantee you as my patient is that during the time left to you, the quality of your life will allow you to live with a sense of dignity and comfort.

I talk to my patients about making the decision to live fully while they're still alive. And I would certainly say that this talk is my biggest, most productive role as a physician. Ironically, it has very little to do with what is taught in medical school. What I do out there with the machines may be excellent, but unless I can inspire my patients to take on a positive attitude, I'm not being very effective. No treatment is worth anything if the patient is worrying all the time about dying.

I've spent a great deal of time thinking about how we can educate people who are preparing for and progressing toward death. I want to guarantee that my patients have really lived.

BRYANT: If only we could begin to realize that dying is as natural as birth, or as natural as living.

BRENNER: I contend that dying is natural only if you've lived first—only if you've lived fully. Of course, everybody who is born must die. What I'm asking is, how do we teach people to live before they die? How do we teach them to be in the moment, to be right now?

If each one of us learned to live with the understanding that life is only one day long, we would live differently. I believe this is the answer, the key to living fully and to dying with some feeling of readiness and contentment. I know I certainly haven't learned this lesson well enough yet, myself.

BRYANT: Your work with cancer patients must raise a number of questions in your mind.

BRENNER: Yes, one of the questions I have, after dealing with death and dying for thirty-five years, is, "What can the living learn from the dying?"

Certainly I've learned that no one is inviolable. Therefore, each one of us should be prepared for the ultimate end that we try to ignore or deny until we are too far down the road. Mostly, we have to understand that every day is a precious thing. There are no guarantees for tomorrow.

BRYANT: You've been able to remain open to your experience, even though it has brought you some pain and frustration. Do you think that most doctors who deal primarily with cancer patients can remain open in this way?

BRENNER: In many cases, physicians do become defensive over the years—not only because of the emotional trauma of losing so many patients, but also because of the threat of malpractice. The fear of malpractice suits forces us to practice medicine defensively. It's had a big effect on the changing orientation of medical care in this country.

BRYANT: How do you feel about some of the changes that have taken place during the last thirty-five years or so?

BRENNER: I'm in favor of private care as opposed to institutional care. I think a strong doctor-patient relationship is extremely beneficial to the patient, because there are many aspects of illness which must be treated, above and beyond what we can accomplish with the physical treatment. Part of this includes developing a personal relationship, transmitting a sense of confidence in the doctor so that when the patient has problems and fears, there is someone to share those fears and problems with, someone who can possibly help to neutralize them for varying periods of time.

Fifty years ago, we had the family practitioner. I remember that as a kid, when the doctor came to see a sick member of the family, we would all rush around, scrubbing the bathroom, putting out the new soap and clean towels. The doctor was treated differently from any other individual who came into the house. He inspired a great deal of respect. We almost imagined an ethereal aura around him. Today, that's not the case. If you sit with almost any group of people socially today, by and large, they talk their doctors down. "Oh, those guys are interested only in money." Or, "Those guys should be sued more."

BRYANT: I just read about a survey that showed doctors to be our number-one professionals as compared with lawyers, dentists, accountants, etc.

BRENNER: Still, the image of today's physician can't match the physician's image twenty-five, fifty years ago, and I think it's going to get worse. I think medicine is moving further and further away from caring, personal relationships.

The old-time physician is gone. More and more, patient care will be delivered by figures who are not identifiable to the patient. He will see a different doctor every day. Giant clinics will provide treatment, and only the very rich will be able to see a private physician.

What can be done? I think it's important that patients demand individual attention. If they don't get it, then let them look elsewhere.

In my opinion, the image of superiority that surrounds most big institutions of cancer care is misleading. Most of the big places leave much to be desired as far as patient care is concerned. I recently had occasion to see a patient who was being cared for by two physicians at one of the biggest cancer centers in the country. The physicians disagreed with each other, and through their lack of communication, the patient suffered a great deal. This is criminal. Individual patients have got to demand high-quality attention in the institutions they choose, or choose different institutions.

BRYANT: How important a role do you feel faith or attitude has in a patient's surviving cancer?

BRENNER: Well, I will say this: there is an unknown factor which makes certain people break all the rules and defy the statistics. For instance, I can see a patient with cancer of the lung, which has metastasized to some other part of the body. Now, nine out of ten people with that condition will be dead in less than a year. But one person with the exact same disease will live two, three, four, five years, maybe longer. Why?

I knew a woman who, after having a breast removed, was perfectly well for twenty-six years. Then suddenly the cancer began to grow once more on her chest wall. Now why did that cancer stay quiescent for twenty-six years, and what made it grow twenty-six years later? Where was it for all that time? This is one of the unknown factors, something we don't understand at all.

Many highly qualified, well respected scientists say that cancer, once it lives and develops, is present in the body. It may never grow again, but it is there. Why does it grow in some? Why does it not grow in others? We simply don't know. These are some of the unknown factors.

One of my patients came here two years ago, with carcinoma of the lung and metastasis to the brain. She's perfectly well today, two years later! Statistically, she should be dead. I'd like to mention that she's a very dynamic lady; she smiles all the time; she doesn't live in fear. Her attitude is superb. Is that just a coincidence?

There are others who, no matter what I say to them, remain acutely depressed. One lady I know went so far as to try to kill herself. She was a bright, wealthy woman, with carcinoma of the breast. She and her husband lived near my home, and I knew her somewhat socially. When she became my patient she said to me,

"When I decide to die, don't interfere," and in response, I said, "Well, that's your prerogative."

About two years later, I got an emergency call from her husband. He'd found her in bed with a bottle of pills next to her, and she was unconscious. He begged me to come over, so I reminded him of the talk we'd had. "Remember that we agreed to let her die when she decided that it was time?" And he said, "Yeah, but I can't do it." So I said, "Well, she may not appreciate it, but I'm a physician, and if you ask me to come, I must." So we pumped her stomach and she came back. Then when I came to see her in her room, where she was lying comfortably cleaned up, she said, "You broke your promise to me. I never want to see you again." And she wouldn't talk to me. She died a few days later.

Now, did that woman's despair hasten her demise? I can't say. I can't tell you that one's emotional state affects longevity. But I can guarantee that attitude and emotional state do affect the quality of life. Attitude can make the difference between a person's feeling crippled by cancer and a person's feeling challenged by it. One will be lying in bed, in misery, while another who is experiencing the same degree of physical pain will get up and go to work each morning. So the answer to your question is that certainly the quality of life is affected by a patient's attitude. But we can't be certain that longevity is affected. It might be.

BRYANT: Do you have any laboratory experience that would support some of your feelings about the importance of attitude?

BRENNER: Yes, actually. In the late 1950s, when I was first starting, I worked with a federally-funded national research group. At that time, I observed something that was very interesting to me. At Maimonides Hospital here in Brooklyn, I was involved in treating ovarian cancer with methotrexate and radiation. That was in 1958. I was impressed with what we were accomplishing; it was the beginning of chemotherapy.

I wrote a national protocol which was used to study ovarian cancer. Around fourteen hospitals contributed to that study. Lo and behold, I found that in no other hospital were the results quite as good as mine, although these were all major hospitals with high-quality physicians. Outside of Maimonides, treatments were actually less effective. If I got two out of five to respond to my treatment program, other physicians got just one out of five to respond. But everyone was using exactly the same treatment. Exactly the same procedures were followed. I came to the conclusion then, that the treatment of cancer was not as simple as one plus one equals two.

For example, I found that in other institutions many more people got sick from the treatments and dropped out of the study. Fewer people would complete the program. So I said to myself, "Why are my patients doing so much better than those receiving exactly the same treatment from other qualified people?" Was it that the others might just have had less enthusiasm about the study? As a result of my own findings, I determined that caring for cancer patients involves more than just giving a person some medicine and seeing what happens. I came to the conclusion then that there is an unknown factor, and that the unknown factor might have something to do with the enthusiasm of the physician—the doctor/patient relationship.

BRYANT: Do you know of scientific studies that would support your conclusion?

BRENNER: Actually, Dr. Carl Simonton, a radiologist/oncologist who was chief of radiation at Travis Air Force Base in California, has done studies in this field. In 1973, he opened a special center for the use of meditation, visualization and psychotherapy, in addition to standard therapy, in the treatment of cancer patients. In one experiment, he took six hundred women with cancer of the breast and divided them into two groups. One group got the standard therapy, period. The other group got the standard therapy, but in addition they also got all kinds of psychic support: emotional, spiritual, psychological. Anyway, that group did, statistically, significantly better in survival than the group that was treated in only a standard fashion.

BRYANT: In Illness as Metaphor, Susan Sontag discusses the danger of associating attitude with the contraction of cancer. If a patient feels responsible for having contracted an illness, he or she may become burdened by a cycle of guilt, which could deepen the emotional problems that go along with having the disease. At the same time, it is important to recognize the effect that attitude has upon our ability to maintain health and encourage the natural healing process.

BRENNER: There are many ways of helping people to feel more positively about themselves. For instance, emotional support is a key factor in treating patients. I don't say that the way I care for my patients actually affects their longevity, but certainly the quality of life among my patients is better than the quality of life of a patient attending a big medical center where each patient is just a number. It's so important to make an effort to sit and talk with patients as individuals, or to be available to them when they have a problem at home, for instance. As a private physician I can do these things. And I would match the progress of any of my patients against a comparable patient at a major medical center where there is no emotional support.

BRYANT: Do you feel that the patient's family plays an important role in creating a structure of emotional support?

BRENNER: Yes. It's very important. It doesn't always happen, but I do invite the patient's children, parents or companions to come and talk with me. I tell my patients that they should have one or two confidants who are aware of the problem so that they can talk with them about it. But I also tell them, "It's not necessary to discuss the fact that you have cancer with Mr. Brown and Mrs. Smith."

Most people in this world are simply not aware of the fact that cancer is curable. They're probably going to say, "Oh, how horrible. You're going to die!" and for the rest of your life they're going to hover over you as if you're dying. That's going to put some awful pressure on you.

BRYANT: Would you say that first of all, cancer patients must accept their cancer?

BRENNER: Without a doubt. And, to take that one step further, if their cancer is in the category that's curable, I give them the statistics. "Breast cancer, stage one, ninety percent rate of cure." I make them walk out of here smiling.

In support of the psychological training that I use, many, many families of dying patients have called me to thank me, even after a member of that family has died, for what I did for their loved ones. The greatest compliment ever paid to me came through a woman whom I treated for two weeks. Her condition was hopeless when we started with her. I remember I saw her on a Friday, and she died on Saturday. On Monday, her husband, an elderly Italian man, came to see me with his daughter. They brought me a bottle of wine to thank me for helping her. What greater compliment can there be for a guy like me who has "failed." I mean she died, but obviously I hadn't really failed, because they loved me for how I took care of her.

BRYANT: It's clear that as a physician, your goals go beyond radiotherapy.

BRENNER: Yes. Eighty percent of my patients die of cancer, but I want very much to help maintain and upgrade the quality of their lives. Because, hell, if you're depressed, you know what happens to the quality of your life. Multiply that depression three-fold, and you can imagine what a person with cancer has to confront. When you take a person who's twenty, thirty-five, fifty years old, who has every need and desire to go on, why, it's unbelievable the depth of depression that some of these people are living with. But you try to correct that. You help them see the life they're living a bit differently.

Let's say a patient has cancer of the prostate with metastatic disease to the bone. It's incurable. He's sixty-two years old, and has a successful business. I say to him, "Listen, this disease will probably shorten your life. Knowing the facts, you have to make your plans." He says, "I want to keep working." Well, fine. Keep working. Or the patient's attitude might be, "Well, if I'm going to die, I want to stop working." But I will not accept someone's choice to stop working so that he can lie in bed and wait to die. I simply will not accept that.

If you have things to do that you can't do while you're working, then stop working and do them. But don't stop working to die. Stop working to live.

BRYANT: The first time I spoke with you, you said something that sparked my interest, and in fact played a big role in my wanting to work with you. You said, "I don't consider myself a scientist, but an artist." Can you elaborate on that?

BRENNER: Yes, I see myself as an artist. My art is the way I construct an aura in which my patients can survive. My philosophy of treatment is based on the quality of life. The physician who is not an artist is interested in only the mechanical factors of his profession: "You need 5,000 rads? We'll give you 200 rads a day for twenty-five days." There'll be no discussion about the quality of life, the dignity of life, the purpose of life. Even though we can't cure all cancer, there are many supportive measures available such as methadone, which is a highly effective pain killer. A man I've been treating for the past few years has diffuse metastasis of prostate cancer. He's hopelessly ill, and wracked with constant pain. I put him on methadone, though, and he called two days ago saying, "I feel great." The cancer has not been altered, but the quality of his life has been. Next time he has a problem, he's going to call me again. So although I can't cure cancer, I can help in many ways. This is the art of my profession.

ON THE NEED FOR EXPLORATION IN THE FIELD OF CANCER ETIOLOGY

BRYANT: How do you perceive the evolution of cancer treatment during the thirty-five years that you've been practicing therapeutic radiology?

BRENNER: Well, one conclusion I've come to is that we're making very little progress. Certainly, since the beginning of the twentieth century, progress in the field of cancer treatment has been the rare exception. Billions of dollars and countless work hours have been expended to achieve something, and nothing has been achieved.

BRYANT: Wait. Just a few weeks ago on the news, The American Cancer Society reported that there is now a fifty percent success rate in treating cancer. That would seem to contradict what you say.

BRENNER: Well, we've made progress in the sense of being able to treat a few forms of cancer successfully: choriocarcinoma, Hodgkin's disease, acute childhood leukemia, breast cancer. And we have managed to make diagnoses earlier, which affects the cure rate in almost all cases. For instance, breast cancer is divided into four stages. Stage four is almost hopeless, but there's close to a ninety percent rate of five-year survival for breast cancer diagnosed and treated in stage one. So if I can give a yearly mammogram to every woman over forty, I will be able to effect a relatively high rate of cure.

But have we affected the incidence of cancer at all? No. Nor have we learned anything new about the disease.

So when I say we've made no progress, I mean we haven't learned to prevent the incidence of cancer at all. We haven't learned what causes cancer to begin with.

BRYANT: If we can't actually believe the statistics we're exposed to on TV, radio and the printed media, what do they actually mean? What can we learn from them?

BRENNER: First of all, the statistics look better than they really are. One reason for this is that skin cancer, with nearly a hundred percent cure rate, is included in the statistics.

But let's examine the facts about the cancers which affect us most dramatically. The cancer which causes the most death in America today is lung cancer. Lung cancer's cure rate is less than ten percent. Then, the most commonly occurring cancers— cancer of the colon, cancer of the breast, and cancer of the prostate, each have a fifty percent cure rate, which is the same as it was forty years ago. And we can cure that fifty percent *only* when we detect the cancers early enough. Even skin cancer's high cure rate has nothing to do with our having learned about the disease. Skin cancer just happens to be very amenable to treatment.

BRYANT: What exactly is meant by "cure rate?" The term seems rather misleading.

BRENNER: In all these cases, we use the word "cure" as if we were making a guarantee. There is no guarantee. When we say "cure," all we're talking about is survival for five years after treatment without a recurrence.

So, what happens if you're a physician dealing with the treatment of cancer? You're really fumbling along in the same way as you did twenty-five years ago. I'm no more capable today than I was then. And I think when I say that, I'm speaking for the quality of care in most major facilities.

BRYANT: Have there been no advances in surgery, radiation and chemotherapy?

BRENNER: Surgery has remained unchanged, except for improved anaesthesia and respiratory maintenance. This means we get fewer operative problems; we can feed intravenously with better medication. New surgical skills have not increased the survival rate, but supportive measures have improved so that there's simply less operative mortality.

In radiation today, instead of working with machines that generate hundreds of thousands of volts, we're using machines that work with multimillion-voltage ranges. A little better: fewer complications, fewer problems for the patient, but cure rate essentially the same.

Chemotherapy is a relatively new field. Where we're going with it, I don't know.

For the most part, success has been the exception.

BRYANT: This lack of progress must be the source of a great deal of professional frustration.

BRENNER: I know I'm not the only one, but speaking for myself, I'm frustrated as hell. To be unable to help people as I would like—to know that my means of therapy and the other accepted means of therapy are hit-and-miss—is terribly frustrating.

I am deeply affected by not knowing how to cure my patients—

watching while, for instance, a sweet, forty-two-year-old woman with
two children and a loving husband dies before her time. Why should
she die now? Why are we not able to help someone like that? Are
we really doing the best we can? I have to ask that question.

I can say quite seriously that although I like my identity as a
doctor, and I like the fiscal rewards, and I like my lifestyle, I would
enthusiastically, even gleefully leave the profession if a "cure" for
cancer were indeed found — without any sense of anger or resent-
ment. Anyone who deals with cancer would be glad to see the disease cured. The frustration of cancer is that we really don't know
what we are doing.

I treat everybody as well as I can. I keep up with the literature.
I keep attuned to everything that is available to my patients. I offer
them every opportunity for proper treatment, and still, more than
half of them die of cancer.

It's a very frustrating thing to go to school for thirty years, to
work for twenty, thirty years, and at the age of sixty not know what
you're doing. Maybe I believe that we're really just not doing the
best we can.

Some of the curative agents we use have very serious effects.
In fact, the treatments being used for some cancers and for Hodgkin's disease may in fact lead to an increased incidence of leukemia. The immune processes that defend us against bacterial
infections are actually destroyed by chemotherapy.

Acute leukemia of childhood had one hundred percent mortality up to 1962. Now fifty percent of those children are living five
years, and twenty-five percent of them are living ten years. But
what's going to happen to these kids when they reach twenty? Are
they going to start getting all kinds of weird diseases?

We now have two new diseases: venereal herpes and AIDS.
Where did they come from? Who knows?

BRYANT: I'd like to get back to your suspicion that "perhaps we
are not doing everything we can." Since billions of dollars are being spent annually for cancer research, what do you think should
be done in order to be more effective?

BRENNER: Doing the best we can depends on our willingness
to go beyond treating the symptoms of cancer. A lot more research
should be aimed at understanding the cause of cancer.

"Etiology" is the word used to describe the process of understanding a disease — understanding its *cause*. For instance, pneumonia
is caused by a pneumococcus bacteria. In order to control pneumonia you don't treat the symptoms; you don't treat the cough

or the temperature or the lung congestion. Instead, you destroy the cause or etiological factor: bacteria. By destroying the bacteria with penicillin, you remove the source of the disease. The patient then recovers, and that's the end of it.

BRYANT: And the etiology of cancer?

BRENNER: We don't yet know how cancer starts, or even what it is. And we're really quite far from knowing how to treat it.

Adenocarcinoma of the endometrium, the lining of the body of the uterus, is treated by removing the entire uterus. If we're fortunate enough to detect the cancer before it spreads outside the body of the uterus, the patient is then "cured" by removal of the uterus. Now, of course, if we remove the site of the problem, the problem is also removed. But what caused uterine cancer in that patient? Nobody knows.

We consider that cancer of the breast is "cured"—if we're fortunate enough to detect it when it is still confined to the breast—when we remove the breast. This treatment may eliminate the spreading of the cancer, but how is that really a cure? We're not removing whatever caused the disease; we're just removing the product of the disease.

Treatments like surgery, radiation, and other means of correcting the end product of a pathology in individual patients may actually get rid of the disease, but only fortuitously, and usually only when the disease has been detected quite early in its development.

Worst of all, we're not creating an environment that will resist the disease in the future. So if the disease progresses one stage beyond that situation and spreads to other organs, we have no more treatments.

BRYANT: It seems logical then to emphasize etiological research.

BRENNER: That's how I see it. In my mind, real evolution or progress will come about when we expend more energy in the direction of learning what causes cancer, so that we can completely remove the factor that produces it. Ironically though, instead of doing basic etiological research, we're spending billions of dollars on stage-three studies: studies of treatments which reduce symptoms. Frankly, I think we're on the wrong track with this. We've got to get back to stage-one studies, so that we can find out what cancer actually is. Is it an immunological problem? Is it caused by some bacterial strain? We haven't even answered the most basic questions about the disease, and yet research funding is rarely allocated for etiological research.

The statistics offer a view of how serious the situation really is. Pancreatic cancer, which we haven't learned to prevent or detect early enough, has a rate of almost one hundred percent fatality. Cancer of the stomach, which we have not yet learned to prevent or detect early, has a ninety-five to ninety-eight percent rate of fatality. And, as I mentioned earlier, cancer of the lung, the number-one killer of all cancers in America, has less than a ten percent cure rate.

Until we have learned how to remove the factor that produces these cancers, we have made not one step forward. We have learned how to remove the disease itself, but only if we catch it early. We may remove cancer before it spreads, but until you learn what causes the cancer to begin with, no progress has been made. As far as I'm concerned, we have not yet taken the first step.

BRYANT: Where does the responsibility actually lie for our failure to understand this disease?

BRENNER: We are all responsible, and of course our government plays a role in it. It's this, simply: in our society, the only treatments that are taken seriously are those which offer quick economic returns. And so prevention of disease is not given a very high priority.

BRYANT: So you think that our lack of progress in understanding cancer is somehow related to economics?

BRENNER: Of course. Economics has a hand in everything. Take smoking. We know that smoking causes lung cancer. Why do we allow the cigarette companies to sell cigarettes? Whose responsibility is it to say, "No cigarettes!" Smoking shortens the life of a human being. Whether it be through cancer or coronary disease, smoking shortens one's life span. We make many harmful drugs illegal; why don't we make smoking illegal? Well, can you imagine how many billions of dollars would be lost by the tobacco industry if we did?

By the same token, we know that caffeine increases the incidence of pancreatic cancer, and most likely contributes heavily to cancer of the bladder and of the prostate. Why don't we make caffeine illegal? Is it the resonsibility of the physician to advance such ideas?

BRYANT: You've mentioned caffeine and tobacco, commonly ingested substances, as agents that help cause cancer. For a moment, let's investigate the foods we eat. A great number of people are proposing that cancer may be prevented through diet.

BRENNER: For good reason. Take colon cancer. In Africa, there is no cancer of the colon. However, the incidence of colon cancer among Africans who have lived in America for just one generation is just as great as it is in the white American community. The theory is that it's the change in diet that does it.

We know as well that women who are overweight have a higher incidence of breast cancer. Jewish women have a higher incidence of breast cancer. We think that a diet rich in red meat and in fat leads to both breast cancer and colon cancer. We can't prove this, but I would certainly say that if we want to prevent colon cancer, we should eat vegetables and bulk material like whole grains that produce rapid passage of food through the digestive tract.

BRYANT: More and more doctors are becoming aware of the effects of diet on health.

BRENNER: But that sort of information is rarely made available to medical students. I certainly wasn't taught that in school. I was taught only that you do a barium enema to diagnose colon cancer; you do a colon section surgically to treat cancer of the colon. And so I've dedicated my whole life to the treatment of cancer, but not to the understanding of it. These are two entirely different things. It just reflects the priorities that have been set up by our system.

Look and see how many courses are offered in nutrition during a four-year medical school program. Why?

BRYANT: It must be a tremendous challenge to effect change in medical priorities and practices.

BRENNER: We're working within a very conservative framework. Let's take practices related to breast cancer, for example. Thirty years ago in the United States, the treatment for breast cancer was radical mastectomy. Radical mastectomy involves removal of the entire breast, including the major and minor pectoral muscles, which extend past the arm pit and up to the shoulder. About twenty lymph nodes are also removed during the process of radical mastectomy. During that time, preferred treatment of breast cancer in Italy, France and England was lumpectomy followed by radiation. Lumpectomy is excision of the tumor itself, leaving the remaining breast intact.

Since the late 1960s, the European concept of lumpectomy has been introduced more and more widely to this country. A study was done at Harvard, under the direction of Dr. Sam Hellman, who is now at Memorial Sloan-Kettering, in which they treated patients of breast cancer in the United States with lumpectomy and radiation. Their results were comparable to those achieved through radical mastectomies at Memorial Sloan-Kettering. Then, after this report came out of the Harvard Breast Group under Dr. Hellman, they began to say that maybe lumpectomy and radiation is as good as radical mastectomy.

So a new approach to treatment of breast cancer *is* being developed in America. Doctors will follow the protocol that is established. But not one step has been taken to show how and why women get breast cancer. How do we prevent breast cancer? Again, we're working on the treatment rather than the source of the disease. Hopefully, soon we will be working to lower the incidence of cancer. Now, that would really make a difference. That would be progress.

Progress in cancer treatment will come about when there are organizations set up to learn about the pathology and etiology of cancer. This is not being done, so cancer will probably increase in incidence every year. That's been the case for thirty-five years, and I have no high hopes that the trend will reverse itself.

It seems that no one wants to take responsibility for change in developing new ways of treating cancer. It's risky working outside the domain of the establishment. Anyone who does that has a very tough struggle, especially in the field of medicine. A scientist who works to understand the disease may find his credibility shrinking. If we are really committed to recognizing and removing the cause of cancer, massive changes are called for—changes in perspective, changes in consciousness, changes in approach.

BRYANT: Suppose researchers began working more widely on etiological research. Do you envision a preventive vaccine as the final result of that sort of research?

BRENNER: Perhaps, but in the case of cancer, we may need more than just one vaccine. What we call cancer may very well be many diseases thrown together. For example, choriocarcinoma—a cancer that affected only pregnant women—had a one hundred percent fatality rate years ago. Then a drug called methotrexate was developed, which cured it. Prior to the development of methotrexate, every woman who got choriocarcinoma died. Then, with the advent of methotrexate, a great number of women were cured. That didn't lead to an understanding of choriocarcinoma; it just led to one therapeutic approach. But methotrexate is practically valueless in treating other cancers. When that drug was developed, everyone thought, "We're on our way." But it works beautifully on only one disease. Then there's the fact that cancer is characterized by the qualities of the individual organ in which it develops. Take squamous-cell cancer. Squamous cells are located in various parts of the body, so you can get squamous-cell cancer of the skin, or of the lung. Squamous-cell cancer of the skin is practically one hundred percent curable. Squamous-cell cancer of the lung, treated properly, has a ten percent cure rate. Therefore, we must understand, we're talking about a mixed bag.

Some cancers affect the count of red and white cells in the body, but many cancers don't affect the bone marrow that way at all. Lymphoma will affect the kind of white cell that's present. Leukemia will, too. But with cancer of the lung, for example, a blood count may come up perfectly normal. Cancers aren't all characterized by any one thing that we know of.

BRYANT: I've heard cancer described as an abnormal condition of the cell itself, while others compare it to a foreign germ that has entered the body.

BRENNER: We don't know for sure. Cancer could conceivably be the result of a bacteria. Ordinarily, a cell matures in a sequential, predictable fashion, very much like the total organism. It's born, it lives for a certain amount of time, and then it dies. A normal cell reproduces in an orderly fashion. A cancer cell, on the other hand, begins to divide in an unpredictable, rampant way. During those periods of rampant division, it loses its characteristics of organization.

Every cell in the lung, for example, has its function, its lifespan and its reproductive pattern. But when it becomes malignant, its reproductive pattern becomes unpredictable, and it produces an abnormal structure—a tumor—within the lung. This tumor may erode blood vessels so that a person begins to cough and spit up blood. It interferes with normal aeration of the lung so that the patient may become short of breath. As a pathologist looks at it under the microscope, the cells of a lung tumor are easily identifiable aberrations. But nobody really knows why cells go wild to begin with.

Ask yourself: Why does a normal human being, raised by a normal mother and father, educated at the typical school, attending appropriate religious services, become a criminal suddenly and begin to break laws? That's what cancer seems to be. Cancer cells are structures raised in a normal environment, which suddenly, inexplicably, become unlawful and unpredictable.

In society, we treat the parallel situation by putting criminals in jail. But have we corrected the problems which cause criminals to come into being? No. That's why our jails are filled and over-crowded. Until we learn how to correct the situations which cause criminal behavior, we will continue to have criminals.

BRYANT: The analogy between cancer treatments and jails taking the place of basic changes in approach to medicine and society is interesting—partly because it points out how big the changes must be in order to re-orient our medical system and our society, but also because, like crime, cancer has become a universal problem.

BRENNER: As a society, though, we don't take the problem very seriously. We believe that we are indestructible and that we can get away with anything. We can build more jails; we can hospitalize more people.

And I end up asking myself over and over the same old question: If we can put people on the moon, why can't we cure our number-one enemy on earth?

Striving for a Gentle Balance

TENZIN GYATSO
THE XIV DALAI LAMA

Temporal and spiritual leader of the Tibetan people, Tenzin Gyat-
so, the XIV Dalai Lama, is widely recognized as an impeccable phi-
losopher, teacher, master of Buddhism, and statesman. In 1959, in
response to the Chinese occupation of Tibet, he and other great la-
mas led over one-hundred-twenty thousand Tibetans to India, Ne-
pal, Bhutan and Sikkim in order to ensure their survival and preserve
their cultural heritage, including the banned practice of Buddhism.

The Dalai Lama, whose name means "Ocean of Wisdom," was
born in 1935 to a peasant family in a small Tibetan village. When
he was two years old, he was found by a delegation sent to find a
successor to the XIII Dalai Lama, who had died three years earlier.
His education, centering on Buddhist philosophy and religion, be-
gan at the age of four, and has involved the memorization and in-
terpretation of thousands of pages of the most important Buddhist
texts.

When he was sixteen, he went to China as the spiritual leader of
Tibet and was greeted by Mao Tse-Tung. Since 1987, in the U.S. alone,
he received the Albert Schweitzer Humanitarian Award, the Raoul
Wallenberg Congressional Human Rights Award, as well as the World
Management Council's Humanitarian Award. He assumed respon-
sibility for the Tibetan government at age twenty, at twenty-five, passed
oral examinations in the traditional fields of mastery: logic and episte-
mology; transcendent ethics; centrist metaphysics; normal, paranor-
mal and abnormal psychology; and monastic ethics. This entitled
him to the degree of Geshe, equivalent to a doctorate, which most
scholars only achieve in their forties. Fully trained in the ritual arts
of Tantra, he is qualified to transmit the initiations and consecra-

tions of all four schools of Tibetan Buddhism.

As the first Dalai Lama exposed to modern Western civilization, he has shown a great interest in the contemporary physical sciences, and stresses the need and importance of learning from both the scientific and spiritual disciplines. His interest in Western technology first manifested in his teens, when he disassembled and reassembled a Packard automobile. Since then he has studied the workings of electronic radar, and meets with physicists and other Western scientists in order to learn about and remain current in the field of physics as well as in other branches of science and technology. He is a close reader of newspapers in English and Hindi, and follows world political events with acute interest. An avid horticulturist, the Dalai Lama also knows thousands of flower species.

The XIV Dalai Lama is greatly committed to the promotion of universal tolerance and compassion, and frequently participates in international dialogues on world peace. In 1989, he received the Nobel Peace Prize.

INTRODUCTION

In October of 1973, while making films at Denmark's TV Workshop, I met the Dalai Lama during his first tour of Europe. Drawn to him through my camera during a time of personal quest for self-improvement and fulfillment, I immediately felt a personal connection. Soon, a level of trust was established, which allowed me to put aside my camera and my ego, and simply listen. It seemed as though he were able to read my thoughts, and his words created an opening in me. Confusion and questions which had gone unanswered for years began to be clarified.

I followed him to India in search of the qualities of mind which I had observed and so admired in him, and in Dharamsala began to seriously study and practice Buddhist meditation. This practice helped me to gradually see and break with old, destructive habit patterns, and I found myself beginning to sense the clarity and calmness of mind which I had been seeking. This experience and the continued example of the Dalai Lama were so powerful that I decided to begin working toward becoming a Buddhist monk. I eventually took the final steps in 1974 and lived as a monk for three years.

My contact with the Dalai Lama during the 1970s laid the groundwork for the work I do today as an artist influenced by Buddhist philosophy and practice.

DIALOGUE

BRYANT: The law of cause and effect is understood in almost every culture. If a farmer plants the seed of a poisonous plant, a poisonous plant will grow. Planting apple seeds will yield an apple tree. But here in the West, we find it easy to ignore the causes of our problems. For instance, most of the money in the field of cancer research goes to treating symptoms, or effects; very little money goes to actually understanding the cause of cancer. As a result, cancer treatments are not as effectual as we would hope, and means of cancer prevention are not common knowledge. Would you comment on this situation?

DALAI LAMA: Of course, with any illness it is most effective to concentrate one's energy upon healing the basic cause. If we know the cause of a disease, we are then capable of preventing it. This is the key. So it is important to find the cause instead of treating the results or symptoms alone.

One reason for the Tibetan medical system's success with so many kinds of illness is that we are trying to *prevent* illness. In my own experience, when I feel really healthy, this is the time to take certain medicines. And at other times, any indication of imbalance, although there may be no clearly defined illness, indicates that a certain preventive medicine should be given to help me obtain balance.

The Tibetan medical system is based on keeping the body in balance. Many things are taken into consideration here: the elements which are found in the body, for instance, and the humors.

You will notice that if two people consume some harmful bacteria or germs, one person may get very sick immediately; another person may not get sick at all, though the same amount of poison entered their bodies. This shows that it takes more than germs to make an illness. Tibetan medicine concentrates on keeping the body strong, in a favorable state, so that it is not vulnerable to disease.

Once the inner condition is perfectly balanced, external germs or bacteria can do less harm. This is one way of concentrating on prevention—of keeping one from getting sick.

BRYANT: In the West, there is a tendency to follow aggressive models of healing—militaristic models. We want to "attack" our diseases, for instance. Many of our treatments have strong side effects, which do great violence to our bodies. Few westerners understand the nurturing and protective aspects of medicine.

DALAI LAMA: Things like diet or exercise for health, even meditation for relaxation, are all reflections of the protective energies.

BRYANT: On a larger scale, how can we go about using those
protective energies in order to help bring a balance into the world?

DALAI LAMA: The only way, I think, is to educate, explain. Ad-
vertise it if you have some money. Of course, it is the basic nature
of all things to have contradictions. Everything holds within itself
the seed of its opposite. As soon as one thing takes over, you have
imbalance. So the ideal we strive for in physical nature is not
offense, but gentle balance. Balance is the only thing there is.

BRYANT: I've learned that in the *Abhidharma*, it is said that the
earth will suffer from imbalance and get sick due to human interference as well as to natural forces. As a result, then, human beings will suffer from many new diseases which we don't know about
yet.

DALAI LAMA: Oh yes. I think that comes especially from the
new chemicals being invented. And when these are more available, new kinds of illness will come.

As described in the *Tantrayana*, there are special relationships
between the internal elements and the external elements. External elements include climatic conditions. These affect the internal elements. This is a Buddhist perspective.

As humans, we are closely related with external elements such
as geographical location, changing seasons, all these things. Of
course, now we have man-made ecological problems to contend
with in highly industrialized countries.

Internal elements include the elements we take into our bodies. It is important to realize that a person who fully controls the
inner elements of body and mind can nearly ignore the effects of
the external elements. So we have interdependence and also in-
dependence.

BRYANT: I have seen a person who was very self-centered, unhappy and disagreeable make complete personality changes when
confronted with cancer. Could you talk about the actual potential
of illness as a vehicle of personal transformation?

DALAI LAMA: In general, all tragedies, including illness, may
seem bad in themselves. But if these events are handled in a certain way, they can be a valuable means of gaining experience and
strength. One may profit from all such conditions.

BRYANT: I've seen that illness can serve as a catalyst for the patient to make actual physical or lifestyle changes, which seem to
be associated with a recovery from the disease. Someone who is
smoking and drinking and not sleeping enough, for instance, makes
some basic lifestyle changes, and these changes contribute to a
recovery.

DALAI LAMA: Yes, many changes can be made. In fact, Tibetan medicine follows three stages in curing illness.

First, without using medicine, we make changes in the environment. The patient may need to be in a cooler place, for instance,
or a hotter place. That is the first stage of cure. If that doesn't work,
then we move on to the second stage of cure—a change in diet,
for instance. In the second stage of treatment, we still do not administer medicine. However, if dietary changes bring no relief, *then*
the patient starts taking medicine. Behavior and diet are both very
important.

Also, one's mental state and activity make a great difference.
There is no doubt about this at all. One's mental attitude always
influences one's health. In some cases, one's mental attitude can
turn a very minor problem into a major, unbearable problem. Equally, one's attitude and behavior are changed when one passes
through a difficult time of illness. Just as one's physical condition
is affected by one's mind, one's mind is affected by one's physical
condition.

BRYANT: It's clear that there's a relationship between one's mental attitude and one's physical well-being. What about the relationship between one's mental attitude and one's karma?

DALAI LAMA: Buddhists explain that karma is the fruit of one's
own actions. And since it is created by one's own actions, any karma, no matter how powerful, can be changed by one's actions as
well.

One's mental attitude may have some connection with previous karma. For example, we may have noticed that, almost effort-
lessly, a certain skill or understanding comes to one, as if
automatically. Buddhists believe that such facility is due to one's
own experience in a previous existence. So, if a person was involved
with killing or something like that in a previous lifetime, killing
might come easy. As a child, such a person might take delight in
killing flies and other small animals, for example.

Karma affects our mental processes and attitudes to an extent.
But in this life, it is up to us to practice mind training to affect

our karma and our own mental attitudes and ways of thinking.

BRYANT: By mind training, do you mean the practice of meditation?

DALAI LAMA: It may take the form of meditation. But mind training may also take the form of virtuous activities such as helping others, or even the practice of analytical thinking—that is, thinking in a disciplined way. But you must realize that thinking is not to be confused with worrying. Worrying is an entirely different thing. If a tragedy has occurred, worrying can make you sick. One of the famous Shantideva quotations says, "If you have a problem and there's a way to overcome it, why worry? And if there's no way to overcome this problem, then worrying will certainly not help."

So the thing is to think, to analyze—not worry. Instead of adding more stress by worrying, think in a different manner.

In Buddhism, we say that if this one particular mistake had not been made, something else would have happened, because we ourselves had already planted the seed for a mishap. It is very important to recognize our own role in the making of mistakes. Blame must never be placed upon another.

BRYANT: On another level then, when we develop technology without regard for human health, the seed for mishap has been planted. That mishap may take the form of a nuclear accident, or it might take the form of illness due to polluted air and water.

DALAI LAMA: Yes. But during this period of time, our difficulties, including accidents and illness, are met with great resources. Today, we benefit from a great many opportunities offered to us through the diversity of the human community.

For instance, we are sharing information about many ways of helping ourselves. Mentally we can help ourselves. In the case of a physical ailment, some practitioners who have developed mental discipline and concentration power may concentrate on the site of pain. If they fully concentrate, the pain will disappear. Whenever severe pain occurs, they simply concentrate totally upon the pain itself.

BRYANT: Do you have a suggestion for people who don't have such a spiritual practice or mental discipline? What do you recommend that they do?

DALAI LAMA: As a human being, you should simply use the mind. Think. Perhaps meditate. Worrying will only bring more suffering. There is absolutely no value in feeling stress or worry. What can it bring?

BRYANT: Western medical practitioners are beginning to recognize the role stress plays in becoming ill and becoming well again. Many people are using visualization techniques to help themselves relax, and some even use these techniques to shrink cancerous tumors or to rid themselves of the tumors completely.

DALAI LAMA: Yes, some people now are using meditations with light, using their imaginations. This can be very helpful, I think— visualizing good things in the place of pain; visualizing light. Sometimes they imagine a solid substance becoming smaller and smaller, lighter and lighter, until it disappears. Sometimes this works. Imagination is effective, just as placebos are effective.

BRYANT: Can you talk more about the relationship between mind and matter in the realm of disease?

DALAI LAMA: That is a big topic, and a difficult one to discuss. First we must define, "What is mind?" There is definitely something there, even if all the physical functions of the body have ceased, because even after these physical functions have stopped, thought may go on. Some people, as a result of long illness, actually experience a short period of death. Then they may come back and are able to describe their experience with death. Such things do happen. Besides, many people actually remember very clearly the lives they have lived previously.

Consciousness is that by which a person knows; consciousness is the instrument of knowing. I feel quite strongly that perhaps in the next century, we may make some important discoveries about consciousness and matter. The truly beneficial practice, the practice leading to most discovery, is not necessarily a religious practice. It may be a yoga practice, or even an ongoing scientific experiment in brain function and memory.

Understanding memory is extremely important. How does the memory function, and what is it? Also, let's learn to understand perception. These skills are needed. These are things we want to understand.

Some scientists and physicists are dividing things so that everything becomes very, very small. This is done with the hope of knowing—the hope of getting objective knowledge. We have identified the smaller divisions like atoms and quarks through quantum physics.

But I believe that until we have more information about consciousness, it is very difficult to speak about matter in accurate terms.

BRYANT: So many people today are recognizing the importance of studying the world within.

DALAI LAMA: Yes, there is a great deal to learn. In the West, Eastern philosophy, especially Buddhist explanations about mind, including information about chakras and special cells, can make a measurable contribution to human knowlege. The Eastern sciences can contribute much to the world's understanding of the relationship between mind and matter. Similarly, in order to know reality fully, some scientific findings are very useful. This is the place where Eastern philosophy and Western science can meet. But much work will have to be done.

BRYANT: What do you see as being the foundation of this work?

DALAI LAMA: Without understanding the nature of consciousness and its different levels, it is very difficult to train consciousness properly. For consciousness is trained through consciousness — not through injection, not through surgery, simply through consciousness. There arc many divisions and levels of consciousness. In order to do away with negative consciousness, we have to develop positive consciousness. The solution to any problem related to consciousness lies in consciousness itself.

It's analogous to the situation of wanting to build some very powerful tool or weapon. In order to make such a powerful thing, one would want to use only the most powerful materials, durable metals and so forth.

Simply, consciousness must be treated through consciousness, by consciousness. Like the saying, "for the people, by the people" — it's that kind of thing. Better consciousness through consciousness. There is no substitute, no other way.

There are many interesting ways of experimenting with consciousness — and many dangerous ways.

BRYANT: So it is important for people who are dealing with matter to develop their consciousness as well. This will help them to use and develop matter more effectively.

DALAI LAMA: I am simply saying that in order to know matter, and to understand why and how the universe came to be here in empty space... we must study. And study involves knowing. Knowing involves consciousness. In order to know matter thoroughly, it is important and necessary to know consciousness too.

It may not be necessary for all scientists to study consciousness as well as their chosen fields of study. But some physicists, I know, are studying very deeply. And the more deeply we research, the more questions arise.

BRYANT: Physicists are discovering that they cannot separate their observations of an event from the event itself—because in observing an event, they change it. They're finding that every time they postulate a new idea about a particle—even if it contradicts a previously proven idea—they can find evidence of that idea being correct. Every time. Some people are beginning to suspect that they are, to some extent, creating reality with consciousness and that consciousness can create matter.

DALAI LAMA: This gives us all the more reason to study consciousness as a science, just as we might study chemistry or physics.

BRYANT: Many scientists are doing research on the effects of various mental states, including meditation, on the physical body.

DALAI LAMA: Some modern doctors and scientists have already accepted certain types of meditation and mental training as a part of their own work. They recognize that consciousness and mind are very powerful in our lives. It is now time to work with this information.

BRYANT: Would you say that, on the ultimate level, there is no separation between matter and mind?

DALAI LAMA: I don't know. Even within Buddhist philosophy there are different theories. Some believe these two things are one. Others believe that they are two separate things. I believe that they are separate.

Living Foods

ANN WIGMORE

When Ann Wigmore was eighteen, gangrene spread through her legs, which had been crushed during an accident. Medical doctors advised amputation, but she chose to use diet as a means of healing herself. Eating only fresh, raw fruits, vegetables and herbs, she cured her legs completely within fifteen months.

Thirty years later, having drifted back toward more ordinary ways of eating, Wigmore was diagnosed as a victim of colon cancer and crippling arthritis. Using her early experience of self-healing as a guide, she began to formulate what has become the Hippocrates Living Foods Plan, based on Hippocrates' own advice: "Let food be thy medicine."

Since 1963, the Hippocrates Institute in Boston has served as a center for learning about and practicing the Living Foods Program. Hundreds of people go to the Institute yearly in hopes that changes in diet, attitude and activity will help to eliminate cancer and other noninfectious health problems, including heart disease, allergies, diabetes, arthritis and hypoglycemia. The program includes activities which encourage increased physical energy, confidence, creativity and enthusiasm for living. In 1986, Ms. Wigmore formed the Ann Wigmore Foundation, also in Boston, where she continues her work of public education and health support.

Ann Wigmore's model of health is described in her books, including Be Your Own Doctor, The Healing Power Within, Why Suffer?, The Sprouting Book and Recipes for Longer Life. Her commitment is to help people realize their full potential as whole, strong and spiritually aware beings.

INTRODUCTION

In preparation for this dialogue, I read Ann Wigmore's literature from cover to cover, and for one month I followed the Hippocrates dietary regime as closely as I could. I'd eliminated all cooked foods, all animal products, caffeine and sugar. During the first two weeks of this experiment, I ate only raw vegetables and fruits, sprouts and carrot-celery juice. Daily I prepared blended sunflower-seed concoctions and sprouted almonds. I began immediately to lose weight, and felt tremendously alert and energetic. I observed that the elimination of oils from my diet also seemed to be correcting chronic health problems. But after two weeks, I felt weak and listless. I called Ann Wigmore, who listened to me describe my condition and then exclaimed, "What do you expect? You're not following the program in a balanced way. You need grains, and you need more oil!" Upon her recommendation I added several foods, including Swedish wasa bread and avocado, and immediately felt stronger.

I sensed that the diet could be extremely valuable in healing by purging excess from the body, and I valued the spiritual implications of getting back to fundamental, "living" nourishment. At the same time, having followed the program incorrectly myself, I was aware of the need for proper monitoring by someone who knew the program thoroughly.

In 1985, upon entering the Hippocrates Institute in Boston, I saw what appeared to be hundreds of trays of sprouts, at various stages of growth. Organic wheat grass, sprouted sunflower, alfalfa and buckwheat are some of the many greens that seemed to fill the building with fresh air as well as nourishment.

Guests at Hippocrates stay for two weeks, during which time they attend lectures, practice physical and spiritual exercises, prepare organic soil, plant seeds, water, and harvest their own food. Several counselors are available to help guests deal with many aspects of their health conditions, including psychological problems.

Upon meeting Ann Wigmore, I was amazed by her youthful verve and enthusiasm which, after my own experience, I associated directly with the diet. Her radiance was reflected in all corners of the Institute through ready smiles and genuine warmth. During my stay, I was made more aware that what I had conceived of as a diet is really much more than that. The Hippocrates program, although not for everyone, is a way of life with potential which reaches beyond the physical realm.

DIALOGUE

BRYANT: Food is a part of our social life. Sharing food is equated with sharing love. Giving food bestows comfort and security. These are pleasures with deep emotional roots, so it's no wonder that the habits we find most difficult to change are those related to diet.

When people with cancer and other life-threatening conditions are instructed by their physicians to eliminate alcohol, tobacco, dairy products, sugar, meat, fried foods, coffee, chocolate and other foods, they often have trouble envisioning a life so deprived.

And yet here at the Hippocrates Institute, you actually have people give up the whole process of cooking.

WIGMORE: The Hippocrates program turns things around for people. Some see it as just another diet, but this program is far more than just eating raw vegetables and fruits. It's really a way of life — psychological and spiritual as well as physical. People who truly understand the balance of this lifestyle may benefit from it for years without ever finding a reason to give it up.

BRYANT: And yet, from what I've observed, a large number of people find it difficult to stick to the program.

WIGMORE: When people use the program as if it were only a diet, they often define it as "just raw foods." But eating any old raw food simply will not do. Today, our soil is fertilized with toxic chemicals; food is picked before its time; vegetables and fruits are sprayed, injected, even irradiated for preservation or for color. These foods don't fit into the balanced program of Living Foods. They can't even be completely digested. All the nutrients are not taken in; poisons are taken in. In these cases, it's no wonder that people crave other foods.

The idea of the Living Foods Program is to introduce into the body not just any raw food, but energy of the highest quality — easily digestible nutrients, full of life.

BRYANT: Let's say I want to start following the program, yet until today I've been eating dairy products, sugar, red meat — what is considered to be the "normal" diet. After a few days of eating only living foods, my body is craving those things...

WIGMORE: Your body may be craving these things, and you may feel unhappy without them, especially psychologically, for a couple of days. I can understand that — you're trying to shake some powerful addictions. You must now be giving to the body the very nutrients whose absence causes the cravings. Otherwise you'll be once again on the roller coaster of addiction, which fills nutritional gaps rather badly.

There is a real need for strength and self-discipline at first, before the elements the body needs have been supplied by living foods. But soon, as the body gets what it needs, these addictions gradually loosen their hold.

BRYANT: During my visit here at Hippocrates, I've felt a strong sense of mutual support among guests and staff alike. The environment here seems to be an important part of the program.

WIGMORE: Yes, here you have a team of people who are working together toward the same end. They're thinking the same ideas. This is essential to the program. We're working to remove toxic conditions and nutritional deficiencies. The first thing we do is to give the body nourishment. Toxemia is automatically eliminated by the body when nourishment replaces missing elements. So most important is our desire and ability to nourish.

Also, when the body receives the nourishment it needs, cravings are eliminated, and we don't tend to eat things which are harmful.

The idea is to supply the missing elements with living food — organically grown, easily digestible nourishment. You have no desire for other things, and you continually enjoy your food more as it becomes completely assimilated as nourishment.

Sadly, everyone is hooked on food today, simply as a pleasurable habit. But that's not how it was intended to be. Food is meant to nourish the body, based on what your body needs. One should eat only when one is hungry. Eating is not something to be done while talking and carrying on with other interests. Eating is a type of meditation. It's replacing what your body needs through communion, in a sense, with the earth.

BRYANT: So the Hippocrates system helps people to replace their addictions with a means of becoming healthy.

WIGMORE: Without question. But it's a process which involves more than just the body. It involves the whole mind as well.

Many people come here on Sunday, and by Thursday they tell me that they look and feel better — that the pain has stopped. This is not merely a result of the physical change, although that is certainly a contributing factor. Most of all, it is due to changes in their minds, which have begun to say, "I'm in control here. I'm not afraid anymore." So they relax, and in great part, that's why the pain stops—because they've relaxed—not because the problem has been completely solved.

BRYANT: One thing I've noticed is that when people abandon red meat, dairy products, white flour and sugar, they experience euphoria at first. The Living Foods regime really seems to affect people deeply. Ironically, they often feel so good that they figure they can get away with going back to their old ways of eating and drinking.

WIGMORE: Well, people have their ups and downs, psychologically. Once people are feeling really well, they have more energy, more ideas. They're happier because they've made changes for the better. At that time, they might decide to have a drink or go back to their old ways of eating. And I don't think there is anything wrong with that kind of experimentation. I think it's very valuable. They should know how different they feel when eating different kinds of foods. That is one way for people to recognize the problem as it shows itself. Everybody is different. Everybody has different needs, and different concepts of what to do with life. That is part of the meditation.

BRYANT: Could you give an overview of the Hippocrates program as a whole?

WIGMORE: First, let's talk about the diet itself. It's most important to have the right balance of intake. I can't overemphasize the importance of taking in just the right nourishment so that there is no need for other foods. Just because someone is eating raw, organic foods, it doesn't mean that the diet is properly balanced. Many people think they're too busy to balance their foods. They forget that this is the basis of the whole plan.

Second, for success with the program I think you have to be open to the aspects that go beyond diet. Here at the Institute, we take care of about twenty people at a time; but we have thirty people on staff. These are nurses, counselors, teachers who teach about the whole, total way of relating to food, to one's self, and to God. So it's not just what people call a "diet." The changes one goes through are more than physical changes. For instance, our counselors have been trained to help remove psychological blockages from as far back perhaps as childhood days. And they help each person to understand that he or she is responsible for everything that happens. Everything comes from within. We stress that continually.

BRYANT: Can you give an example of how you get these ideas across?

WIGMORE: Let's say a woman comes in feeling sorry for herself, crying that everything is wrong in her life. Well, instead of letting her cry—because although I think it is very nice to be sympathetic, that would not solve any problem at all—our approach would be to try to awaken her, saying, "You are responsible. While you're involved in your self-pity, how can anything happen differently for you? Shape up. Begin to think about what you really want and need. Then things will begin to open up for you." Because as long as she interprets everything that happens to her as being negative, every person she meets will contribute to that negativity somehow.

BRYANT: So you approach the problem of negative attitude as part of your program.

WIGMORE: Yes, but we're not on an assembly line here. Everyone has different needs. Everyone who gets involved with the diet is also involved with an evolving, personal education. This program is not one, unchanging plan. In fact, to my mind, that's the problem with medical science, and with the world of organized religion. They want to give a prescription once and for all—just one answer for everyone. A label. It isn't surprising to me that our outdated political and religious structures are losing their ability to function positively in people's lives.

This will only change when people begin to know themselves, and when they find ways of integrating all the parts of themselves, fully recognizing the God within.

BRYANT: It seems that you're helping people to integrate the intellectual, emotional and spiritual aspects of their healing process with the physical changes taking place in their bodies. How do you see the Hippocrates program as fitting into the holistic health system?

WIGMORE: Of course we're a holistic center, but I don't like to use the word "holistic" because it's so misunderstood today. Many people who call themselves holistic therapists— those who work with vitamins, for instance—use hit-and-miss methods to treat symptoms. Well, how can we tell for sure whether a certain organ needs a particular vitamin or mineral to function properly? And if we do know that the kidneys need a certain vitamin, how could we be sure that when that substance goes through the bloodstream, the kidneys will make use of it fully?

The people involved in administering vitamins and other types of therapy could be a marvelous force for helping people right now, if only they would stop "treating" specific symptoms and just allow the body to establish its own strength through proper nourishment.

There are no two bodies alike on this planet, so diagnosis and treatment are a lot more complex than most people understand. It's best to offer the body a type of nourishment which is already perfectly balanced, and which can easily be taken into the bloodstream to benefit all of the body at once.

BRYANT: While the complete Hippocrates program might be ideal for someone dealing with an acute health problem, I'd like you to address the people who are apparently healthy. How can one gradually work toward practicing the principles of your program?

WIGMORE. The only way to begin is by giving the body better nourishment. By this I mean eating more and more living foods: sprouts, seeds, organically grown fresh fruits and vegetables. It's important to eliminate all drugs, including caffeine, and to eliminate all refined foods, especially sugar and white flour, since they rob the body of enzymes without adding nutrition. Meat should also be removed from the diet. If these steps are followed, not only the body but the mind will improve greatly.

People can make these changes at home successfully, although some of them are difficult to make in the everyday home environment, around the refrigerator—around the old habits. Often it's the most acutely ill people who have the strongest desire to make the necessary changes. And most often, these people have the greatest success.

BRYANT: So someone with bad eating habits can eliminate them one by one, slowly...

WIGMORE: Whatever our bad habits are, they must be eliminated if we want well-being. We're talking about survival here. At the Institute, we're extremely strict because we want quick results. How can people go on a transitional diet—for instance, still eating cooked foods—when their lives are threatened by cancer? There isn't time. If you really want to do it, your mind will carry you through. There is absolutely nothing to stop you. It's a matter of decision.

BRYANT: But the people who have the motivation to do it are a rare exception.

WIGMORE: This program is not for everyone, but it will give you another chance at life if you want to live badly enough and if you're prepared to make the changes you need to make. It *is* possible to recover your health.

BRYANT: How successful has your program been for cancer patients? Is simply following the program sufficient to cause remission of most cancers?

WIGMORE: About eighty percent of our guests have cancer, and I have never seen a failure. By that I mean that everybody responds. Response is natural. But in order to fully succeed, a person must activate certain qualities.

First, desire. A person must have a great desire for success. But desire is only the planting of the seed. If it is to grow, there is a need for action. Reading one hundred books won't help you unless you're really willing to do something about your condition. Here we have people learn by doing. People help themselves so that the method becomes a part of their lives. This is a requirement for success.

Also, there must be a willingness to explore emotions. So we have an entire program of emotional support, with counselors who have been trained to deal with the fears and questions that come up with such changes.

And the results we look forward to are better than remission. When we introduce the Living Foods lifestyle, we say that the body is healing itself by eliminating the cause of cancer. There is a big difference between this and remission.

BRYANT: If the Hippocrates diet actually works to eliminate the cause of cancer, why is it that people who go back to "normal" food often get relapses of their condition?

WIGMORE: You can't expect the body to keep you healthy after you go back to the thing that caused your cancer in the first place.

I can't guess what will happen to people who leave the program, so I don't call this method a cure. It's an ongoing program of living, and it's nothing terribly new. It's just turning back to nature's way, and the way of nature is growth—spiritual growth.

BRYANT: Can you speak about how you see cancer and its evolution in our society?

WIGMORE: Well, first I ask, what is cancer, anyway? Physical imbalances become cancer little by little, in stages. It's not that cancer hits you all of a sudden. It's a matter of cells dying, decaying and not leaving the body. First you have colds, fever, tumor — these are warnings. These warnings, due to deficiency and toxemia, are given in order that we might do something about the problem. It's the body's way of saying, "If you don't do something about your health, you're going to get something more serious." On the other hand, if you treat the symptoms themselves without changing the condition that caused those symptoms, another set of symptoms will take over, also as a reminder for you to deal with the problem being presented to you.

BRYANT: What kind of research have you done to determine that cancer is a gradual process?

WIGMORE: I just finished a research project on live blood cells, and I'm very interested to see whether others will pick up on this work. Very simply, it involved watching blood cells and observing the effects of different kinds of nutrition on those blood cells. Twenty people participated.

You take a small amount of blood from a person and you put it under a microscope. Greatly magnified, that image is then projected onto a television screen, where you can observe the cells and see exactly what they're doing. It's interesting to see that cells nourished in different ways exhibit entirely different orders of activity.

During the experiment, one very healthy, intelligent young fellow was called to register for the army. In order to avoid being recruited, he started eating a lot of sugared dairy products, which immediately affected his feeling of well-being. But the most interesting thing is that the pollutants could be seen on the screen. Within just two weeks, his blood cells showed great abnormalities. And he had been a basically healthy person.

BRYANT: Doesn't the body's own defense system protect against such abnormal changes?

WIGMORE: Of course we all have defense systems, but we overwhelm them habitually, so they're not working at optimal capacity. For that reason, so many of our modern habits are dangerous—overeating, for instance—because the minute you put something into the body, all kinds of things start happening. But even more important than the contents and quality of the food you take in, the state of your mind should be taken into consideration. Are you under emotional stress? Of course, eating the wrong foods can put you under great physical and even emotional stress.

All of these things affect our natural immune systems.

BRYANT: So many people today are working with natural substances in new ways, either as alternatives or to complement conventional medical therapy. As you mentioned earlier, some administer vitamins and even minerals in megadoses. Others may replace single, needed elements in the body. Can you talk more about some of these methods of supplementing the body with what it seems to need most?

WIGMORE: Those methods are entirely different from what we're doing here. We want to offer the body complete foods. The body's balance must come from the balance which already exists in whole foods. It does not come from taking large doses of single things that the body needs. The body only needs single elements when the food it has taken in is not balanced food.

The problem is that the scientist, in general, tries to manipulate nature, but does not understand nature. The most scientific, the most effective medicine comes directly from nature, and not in vitamin or medicine bottles. Giving somebody one specific element or chemical is not in nature's plan, because no food in nature has only one ingredient. Nothing is pure in nature. So how can a single element be optimal for the body?

Think about vitamins for one moment. Vitamins are a life force. Can the life force actually be preserved in bottles? When you juice a fruit or vegetable, about one half-hour later, the vitamins are gone — because they're part of the life force. How can the life force ever be preserved?

Ideally, the cells should take in nourishment which is already balanced. That's nature's way of doing things. And in being more balanced, plant food is much more efficient than animal food. Even the U.S. Department of Agriculture admits that the human body uses about eighty-nine percent of the protein offered by sunflower seeds, whereas we can use only about thirty percent of the protein found in meat. So chances are that meat will be generating far more pollutants in the body, because the nutrients are not all assimilated. Meat is not a well-balanced food in itself.

You can grow four hundred pounds of protein from grain seeds on just one acre of land. In contrast, raising flesh food, we get just forty pounds of usable protein on that same acre of land. Especially shameful is the fact that the earth is used for an industry of killing, because killing on any level is the very thing that destroys our harmony. It's this loss of our harmony that causes dis-

ease or poverty and war. And animals are so important... how can
we be killing them when we don't need to? It goes against the laws
of nature.

From just one pound of seed you can grow ten to twelve pounds
of sprouts. We could increase the value and volume of our food
chain tremendously, while using our land as nature intended.

BRYANT: How do you see the future of the Living Foods movement? Is it likely to be a household topic for discussion, say in the
next five or ten years?

WIGMORE: I think the future is very bright, although in general, conditions for living are very bad. We're facing some grave problems here on this earth. As a result, people are waking up; people
are becoming more aware, and are beginning to understand the
need for spirituality.

Sometimes people are afraid to move toward things which represent change, even if the change might be very helpful to them.
But basically, I see that many, many people are moving in ways
that help to clarify our relationship with the earth. I hope and pray
that we can interest more and more people in really feeling concern for reaching this balanced relationship with nature. Nourishment is the key, and the earth offers us that nourishment.

BRYANT: Can you talk about any specific lesson that cancer may
have to teach us?

WIGMORE: I think that one reason cancer is so widespread is
that so many people today are ignoring, violating, misinterpreting,
and misusing the laws of nature, which are actually designed to
bring us toward harmonious living. I think the many spiritual pathways are helpful in furthering the natural law.

But even the most wonderful spiritual pathway is missing something very important if it does not take into account how the body
is nourished. All people who recognize how the spiritual energy
within themselves can be a guide should have a good understanding about how energy in the form of food affects the whole human being.

The body's basic nourishment is the energy that comes from the
Earth. We understand so little of the Earth, so we disregard it and
waste many of its gifts — even though we know that without these
gifts, our bodies couldn't even function. Without communication
with the Earth and attunement with it, why live on this Earth? If
the Earth is misunderstood and wasted, if land and nourishment

meant to be used are not well utilized, then even the most beautiful, spiritual people suffer ill effects.

BRYANT: So many people who live by spiritual values are working gradually toward what they believe to be the ideal state. But the customs of today's society—not only cooking food, but eating sweets or prepared food, and taking caffeine, alcohol and other drugs, for instance—influence us strongly.

WIGMORE: Why be held back by the customs of society when we're supposed to be working from within ourselves? When customs are based on looking outside of ourselves for the answers, we can lose out by following blindly. In fact, we can easily destroy the very things we want—especially the energy that allows us to work toward a better world.

For instance, I must have a living garden in the kitchen. Well, the conventional, physical rule is that you can't have a farm on the fourth floor in the city. But letting my own inner voice show how, I break with conditioning and make the changes that are needed in my life.

BRYANT: Surely you've seen a raising of consciousness about diet during the last ten years or so.

WIGMORE: There's no question about that. But how many people realize that what's needed is simply to remove the cause of illness—to give the body a healthy environment, and become strong and healthy again? That's all there is to it. There is no "cure." There is simply a chance to remove the cause of illness, to give the body a chance to become healthy, and to heal itself. Everything is there; everything comes from within.

BRYANT: You came to an understanding of the Living Foods pathway through an illness of your own. Could you talk about the potential value of illness?

WIGMORE: Yes, my own health problems brought me to this, and I personally believe that health problems can be the greatest blessing in the world, if you want to live for a long time. I was completely old at fifty. My hair was gray, and I could only work for about two hours a day. Now I'm going on 78, and I work all day, every day, sleeping about one or two hours total, maybe three. My body can handle this because I listen to my inner voice. I'm aware of what I have to do. Everything comes from within.

I benefited from my own illness, and everyone has the ability to do this. We have that free choice. But we have to be quiet and calm in order to make decisions. We can't be looking around to see what everyone else is doing. We have to listen to our inner voices to learn, to make progress and to grow through experience. We all have to understand ourselves. Then we can make the changes we want to make.

Working Within The System

ARTHUR C. UPTON, M.D.

Dr. Arthur Upton, director of New York University's Institute of Environmental Medicine, has been involved in researching the effects of radiation and other environmental factors on human beings since 1951.

He began working in the field of radiation injury at the Oak Ridge National Laboratory in Tennessee. During his eighteen years there, he contributed to long-term research studies which have contributed greatly to international understanding of how radiation acts.

Subsequently, Upton worked for seven years as chairman of the Pathology Department at the State University of New York at Stony Brook (1969-77). From 1977-80, he served as director of the National Cancer Institute before accepting an invitation to become chairman of the Institute of Environmental Medicine at New York University. The Institute sponsors etiological research on environmentally related diseases, with the ultimate goal of preventing such diseases.

INTRODUCTION

During my meetings with Dr. Arthur Upton, I came to know a man who is not only generous with his time and energy, but also highly expressive. His commitment to education was evident as he took time from his very demanding schedule to share knowledge and perspective gained from years of scientific research and administrative service. Although Dr. Upton said he was not a "deeply philosophical person," his personal integrity and sense of justice made a tremendous impression on me. This humble human being is indeed a philosopher — a deeply and ethically concerned individual.

My exchange with Dr. Upton, who is a dedicated research scientist and pillar of the medical community, dissolved any stereotyped attitudes or ideas I may have had about the "ivory tower" of the scientific world.

DIALOGUE

A PROFESSIONAL HISTORY

BRYANT: What caused you to choose a life of work in the cancer field?

UPTON: I embarked on a career in medicine, and after I was well into my internship and residency, decided that research would be more in keeping with my personality and goals than a career in the practice of medicine. So I went into pathology to study the causes of disease. As I was finishing my residency and aiming at a career in research, an invitation came from Drs. Jacob and Olga Furth, great experimental pathologists, to join them at the Oak Ridge National Laboratory in Tennessee.

Back in the early '50s this was a tremendous windfall, because there were very few positions for anyone in pathology, or in any branch of medicine, that allowed for full-time research. Research was something you had to squeeze in at the end of the day or on weekends. So I joined the Furths at Oak Ridge and became immediately involved in the study of radiation injury.

Cancer was the first serious problem I approached. We studied the late effects of full-body radiation on mice. Various cancers developed as a result of the radiation exposure. Our task was to determine what kind of cancers developed in response to what kind of radiation, and when and why they developed. What was happening? What was the radiation doing to produce this response?

BRYANT: Were these rare or special types of cancer you observed in response to radiation exposure?

UPTON: No, that was interesting—these were not unique cancers at all. They were simply more of the same cancers that would have appeared anyway.

BRYANT: How did you determine that it was actually radiation that was responsible for the increased cancer?

UPTON: In general, we found that the larger the radiation dose, the greater the incidence of cancer. This allowed us to conclude that radiation at least does something to stimulate cancer, which might be caused by other variables.

The question was, what is this process? What does it mean? Why is it happening? What is radiation actually doing to modify the frequency of cancer?

I've been at it now for thirty years or more, searching for answers, starting with radiation but also investigating the process of
cancer arising from other causes such as drugs and diet.

It became a very absorbing intellectual puzzle. I found myself
completely immersed in the scientific questions. Then there was
the satisfaction of knowing that the answers, as they became available, might be of benefit to people all over the world. We were working with cancer, a serious problem for humankind. We were
conscious that if we could solve the problem, people would be much
better off.

BRYANT: Those experiments at Oak Ridge created a basis from
which thousands of others could continue cancer research.

UPTON: The work that I did personally, the work that I shared
with the Furths, and the work that I've done with others in succeeding years has been useful in directing other research and in
shaping our ideas as to the way radiation acts. I think it's been important work.

BRYANT: After leaving Oak Ridge, what was your next work commitment?

UPTON: Well, from the time I went into medical school, I had
always intended to become a teacher. I wanted to take part in helping to train and involve young people in the work of understanding the prevention and treatment of disease.

Though I enjoyed doing long-term research concerned with cancer in animals, I eventually took an opportunity to become chairman of pathology at the brand-new Health Sciences Center at the
State University of New York at Stony Brook in 1969. As the dean
of basic sciences, I helped to build a new department from scratch.
It was very exciting, very creative.

The setting at Stony Brook seemed opportune, half-way between
the Brookhaven National Laboratory, which was an excellent radiation research institution, and the Cold Spring Harbor Laboratory, which was strong in molecular biology and genetics. This was
especially attractive because my own research had led me toward
that kind of approach: the role of viral genes, or oncogenes, in car-
cinogenesis.

So Stony Brook seemed good for many reasons. When I got there,
though, it became clear that I would not be able to spend any time
doing the research I had hoped to do. In 1977, when the fun of
building the programs themselves was past, I decided to accept
the challenging invitation to become director of the National Can-

cer Institute at the National Institutes of Health.

I really didn't foresee that the work at NCI would involve quite so much administration and politics, and so little science. As director, it was impossible to devote much time to reading, staying abreast of my field, or interacting with colleagues. My work there was important, but it was about eighty percent politics, fifteen percent administration, and less than five percent science.

It's just the nature of such a big program. The National Cancer Institute, when I was there, had a budget of close to $1 billion a year, a staff of two thousand people, and research support all over the world. It was my job to keep track of the entire program, day in and day out, with the innumerable problems that arose. It involved testifying before different congressional committees every other week or so. But though it was tremendously exciting, and I had opportunities to shape major policies, there just wasn't time to get deeply involved in any particular scientific problem.

So when I was approached to come here as chairman of the Institute of Environmental Medicine at New York University Medical School, I decided to come back to academic life. That was in January, 1980.

BRYANT: Can you describe the purpose of the Institute of Environmental Medicine?

UPTON: Our purposes are: one, to conduct research into the causes of environmentally related disease; two, to train physicians, other health professionals and graduate students in the field so that they can explore and explain the causes of environmentally linked disease; and three, to enable the prevention of such diseases.

Of course, prevention is our ultimate goal.

BRYANT: It seems to me that any approach to medicine that includes environment would have to deal with all aspects of one's surroundings, and not just specific carcinogenic substances. Is that the Institute's approach?

UPTON: Environmental medicine involves more than toxic chemicals or radiation and pollution. We see environmental medicine very broadly, as something that embraces everything that isn't inherited.

This includes the way we choose to live, the lifestyle we adopt, the foods we eat, our smoking or drinking habits, and our sexual practices. All of these external factors that act on our bodies, or on the cells of our bodies, may determine whether we will have a long and healthy life or suffer some disability or disease.

BRYANT: Does your research take the human psyche or psychological factors into account?

UPTON: We are not involved with emotions as such. We haven't gotten into psychology or psychiatry—the emotional stresses.

BRYANT: Would you agree that stress plays an important role in whether a disease like cancer takes hold or not?

UPTON: Yes, stress is thought to be an important factor in disease promotion and prevention. In our experiments and epidemiological studies, we try to control the possible influence of emotional stress.

BRYANT: How is that done?

UPTON: Well, for instance, we ensure that the environments our laboratory animals live in are essentially the same except for the particular physical or chemical agent that is being introduced.

Let's say we try an experiment in which some animals are exposed to high dosages of benzene; other animals are exposed to moderate dosages; others are exposed to small dosages; some animals are exposed to no benzene at all. We're anxious to determine whether changing the amount of benzene in the inhaled air affects the animals' health, or whether the animal is able to perform as well in a behavioral test, eat as well, live as long, or develop cancer or other diseases as a result of exposure to benzene.

In such an experiment, we would modify the benzene level and try to keep everything else identical. If the animals were housed in different kinds of cages, if population density were different, if males and females were mixed in some cages and not in others— these are factors that might affect the animals' emotional outook. These psychic variables might confound the effects of benzene. The experiment is designed to eliminate such confounding factors.

BRYANT: Are you able to experiment in a similar way with human beings?

UPTON: If we were looking at the effects of benzene or lead or other external factors on human populations, we would first make every effort to determine whether the incidence of socioeconomic problems, broken marriages, or other sources of emotional stress varied among groups. If so, we would try to structure the population groups that we were comparing so as to neutralize those differences. That way, factors that could confound the analysis would be recognized and properly controlled in the design. But, though we recognize the role of stress as an environmental variable, we haven't looked into it systematically. It's not that stress and other psychological factors aren't important, it's just an area we haven't pursued.

On the other hand, we're doing research in the fields of neurotoxicology and behavioral toxicology. These studies involve research on stimuli that affect behaviors, such as feeding patterns, general activity patterns, ability to learn, and ability to perform learned tasks.

BRYANT: Can you give an example of behavioral toxicology?

UPTON: You teach a pigeon, let's say, to push a certain button to gain an item of food, and the pigeon learns that it has to push the button swiftly three or four times to get the reward. Then you expose the pigeon to a very low concentration of benzene. You may find that before the pigeon shows any other manifestations of toxicity, it loses proficiency at rewarding itself; it forgets how to push the button, or it can't push the button fast enough. Clearly, in such a case, we have evidence that behavior is being affected by the substance we've introduced. That's the kind of measurement we're dealing with.

BRYANT: And what is meant by neurotoxicology?

UPTON: Neurotoxicology denotes damage to the nervous system—one of the most serious effects of lead poisoning, for instance. There is evidence now that children who are exposed to lead early in life develop a deficit of intelligence. Children with high blood-lead levels starting early in life don't score so well on IQ tests. We now know that *any* increase in blood-lead will cause some decrease in psychometric score. There may be no absolutely safe level. So we're concerned about how external agents, including chemicals, may affect intelligence, the nervous system and behavior.

BRYANT: You're also involved with industrial or occupational medicine, which has more to do with the hazardous effects of working conditions. Am I right?

UPTON: Yes, we have a program in industrial hygiene, which includes ergonomics. This involves the designing of people's working and living environments, as well as equipment used during work and at home, so that they're conducive to enjoyable, effective performance.

BRYANT: I'm especially interested in your work at Oak Ridge, not only because of the way it has affected science, but also because it was an outgrowth of the Manhattan Project, which led to the development of the atom bomb. Could you speak about that work?

UPTON: The Oak Ridge Laboratory was designed as a military effort, but it soon became apparent that atomic energy had peaceful as well as military applications. In harnessing the atom for human betterment, many problematic aspects were examined closely — such as how to build reactors that would operate safely and efficiently, and how to protect people and the environment. Different kinds of studies were undertaken to help regulate against overheating and meltdown, or escape of radioactive material into the environment.

For many years since then, the Department of Energy has spent $100 million a year or more to study the effects of radiation, including risks to the population. But the Department of Energy is just now looking at its worker populations in all of its big laboratories: Oak Ridge, Los Alamos, Hanford, and so on. This kind of study should be continued.

BRYANT: Since radiation seems to be a major stimulus involved with contracting cancer, it strikes me as paradoxical that it's also used in cancer treatment. When was radiation first applied as a therapeutic measure?

UPTON: A German scientist named Roentgen discovered the x-ray in 1895. Within just a couple of years, x-ray machines were set up all over the world to treat people with cancer. So we've had ninety years to study how radiation might be used to treat cancer. At the same time that radiation was observed to be useful in medical diagnosis and treatment, it was also observed to cause injury.

In the early days, radiologists burned their own fingers, literally; and they sometimes overtreated their patients and made their patients ill.

BRYANT: So people discovered that radiation is a double-edged sword. You can do good with it; you can also do harm.

UPTON: Yes, and in order to do good with it, you have to avoid doing harm. The laboratory at Oak Ridge is really an outgrowth of the study of radiation injury, not so much radiation treatment per se. We were concerned with the harm. How does radiation harm cells? How can we prevent harm? Not, "How can we cure cancer, and how can we more effectively treat cancer?"

CHALLENGES IN CANCER RESEARCH

BRYANT: How *does* radiation actually affect cells? What are the physical phenomena involved?

UPTON: We don't have complete knowledge there, but we can see that radiation breaks chromosomes, which are the threads upon which the genes appear to be lined up like beads. If we irradiate cells and then examine them microscopically, we can see that the chromosomes are broken.

Chromosomes can actually be shattered. If two chromosomes are broken side by side, the breaking point of one chromosome may be healed and reunited with the breaking point of another chromosome, giving rise to chromosomal rearrangements. These can alter the cell.

We can measure genetic changes—mutation resulting from exposure to radiation. In the laboratory, we see these results in proportion to dose, down to the smallest doses that can be studied. It's possible that these mutations continue to occur in proportion to dosage all the way down to the *slightest* amount of radiation—what we call natural background. I think that these damaging effects on chromosomes and genes are probably the most important kind of radiation injury that occurs.

BRYANT: Does radiation injure other parts of the cell as well?

UPTON: There's no reason to think that radiation doesn't damage other parts of the cell. But it doesn't have the same effect if it breaks a water molecule, for instance, because in that case, billions of other water molecules will remain intact. On the other hand, if the cell loses one gene, there may be no other one quite like it. The cell may need that one gene to remain normal, and to reproduce normally. If that one gene is damaged with radiation, the cell itself may be damaged irreparably.

BRYANT: When we're exposed to radiation, do genetic changes occur immediately, or after a specific amount of time?

UPTON: They take place at once. Damage to the cell may occur within a matter of minutes, or hours. But this damage may not express itself for a long time. A-bomb survivors are getting cancer now in increasing numbers, forty years after the bombs were dropped. The cancers of many of these people are directly related to that radiation exposure.

BRYANT: So there may be a long period of inactivity before the cancer actually shows up.

UPTON: Yes. If a mutation or chromosomal change is made in a germ cell of the testes or an ovary, the changes may not be noticed until decades later when the individual has a child. Or the effect of radiation exposure may only be noticed in subsequent generations, when the exposed person's children or grandchildren are born with genetic defects related to the exposure.

Luckily, in Japan, studies done on survivors have not revealed any clear-cut increase in genetic disease. This suggests that these genetic lesions are fairly rare.

BRYANT: Why does it take so long for the effects of radiation to appear?

UPTON: We suspect that the cell or cells from which the cancers arise were altered at the time of radiation, but not enough to start growing at that time. It took other stimuli to bring about disease.

BRYANT: Do you think the process might have something to do with aging?

UPTON: It might. Women who were exposed to the atomic bomb as children are just now developing breast cancer forty years later, while their mothers, who were exposed as adults, showed an increased rate of cancer within five or ten years after exposure. So while it could be just a matter of time, we reason that cancer in the breast also requires hormonal stimulation. Experiments with animals argue that hormonal stimulation *is* required to cause some cancers to grow.

We believe that radiation damaged the cells in those little girls, and that the damage just sat there until they reached the reproductive age, when there was hormonal stimulation of the breast tissue. Only then did the tumor begin to grow and evolve into a clinically discernible cancer. So in cancer biology, we talk about cancer initiation—those changes that occur at the time of exposure—and then those subsequent changes that take place months, years or decades later, involving the promotion and progression of the lesion. We don't know too much yet about these initiation steps. We think they have to do with damaged DNA or genes, but the later steps may involve processes which are yet to be determined.

BRYANT: Much of the scientific information we have now about radiation seems to be closely related to what you learned during the long-term studies you were involved with at Oak Ridge.

UPTON: Yes, back in the 1930s, Jacob and Olga Furth were among the first to observe that after being exposed to x-rays, mice develop leukemia in increased frequency. Depending on the type of leukemia and the radiation dose, you might see some leukemia within six months, but the major effects occur somewhere between the first and second year. They were among the first to see this, and they continued to study the problem. I joined the Furths in '51, fifteen years after their initial observations. They were deeply concerned with the nature of this effect.

What *was* leukemia? Was it a cancer? If so, how did radiation injury trigger the production of this disease? In studying leukemia, it became obvious that it wasn't the only kind of cancer that was induced by irradiation.

So when I arrived, a number of experiments had already been set up to determine the different kinds of tumors that would occur, and to explore how they came about.

BRYANT: You were interested in understanding the precise relationship between cancer and radiation exposure?

UPTON: Yes. We wanted to know whether the risk of cancer was simply proportional to the exposure, or whether there was some range of doses, somewhere at the lower end of the dosage scale, where no effects at all occurred. Was there a safe level? What if you spread the dose out over a period of time? What if, instead of giving a whole dose in a few minutes, you administered it over a few days, or a few months, or spread it out over the animal's entire lifetime?

We can speak about most poisons, alcohol among them. If you were to take a drop of alcohol in a teaspoon, once a day every day of your life, you probably would see no effect at all. You would then have taken more than a quart of alcohol over an entire lifetime. But if you sat down today and drank that entire quart at one time, you'd be dead tomorrow, or at least terribly sick. So with alcohol, spreading a dosage out over a long period of time eliminates its toxicity.

We wanted to find out whether, if we spread the dosage of radiation out over time, we would eliminate its toxicity. Would cancer simply not show up under these circumstances? These were the kinds of experiments we were doing.

BRYANT: Experiments which were obviously very important for human safety.

UPTON: Yes, because, for instance, if nuclear energy is going to be useful to society, there will be a general increase in the levels of radiation to which everyone is exposed. Does this automatically translate into more cancers and other effects? And if so, what are the risks? Those were our questions.

In our research, we were actually concerned with distribution of the radiation dose throughout the body and throughout the cell. If we were to irradiate only a particular organ like the breast, would we get cancer in other areas which were not exposed, such as the kidney? Was risk a function of the number of cells which were irradiated? If we irradiated half an organ, would we have only half as much risk as if we'd irradiated the entire organ?

BRYANT: And what did you find?

UPTON: We found that if you irradiate the breast, exposure may cause a severe breakdown of breast tissue. If the dose is smaller, you may see no immediate signs of injury; but decades later, the breast may develop a cancer which would not otherwise have occurred, as we've seen in the case of women who were exposed as children. As far as we know, the effect of radiation is limited to the area of exposure.

If we irradiate the big toe, we won't produce a breast cancer. Irradiating any other part of the body doesn't seem to cause breast cancer. Only irradiating the breast does that. But as I said earlier, any amount of radiation exposure may cause some changes which could be damaging in ways we may not be able to detect for generations.

BRYANT: Does this support the theory that it's the irradiated genes which are responsible for cancer?

UPTON: Our research did support that theory, yes. We became persuaded that the most sensitive part of the cell was the gene, or the genome—the genetic material. We then concluded that the resulting carcinogenic effects are in all likelihood related to some sort of radiation damage or change in the genes of the cell.

We found that we could grind up tumor tissue, make a cell-free filtrate, and in some cases, transmit the cancers by cell-free material. And this was consistent with our belief that, in this case, the cell-free filtrate was the source of the altered genes. The genes were responsible. Today we are fascinated with the oncogenes. We wonder how radiation activates those oncogenes.

BRYANT: One of the things I have a hard time understanding is why twentieth century Americans choose to live with radiation in increasing amounts. We know the risks, but growing numbers of people want radiation-emitting items like microwave ovens and word-processors. Most recently, irradiated foods have been introduced to increase shelf life. We've chosen to work with a source of power that is inherently hazardous, and there doesn't seem to be an end in sight.

Instead of looking for non-radiation-producing technologies, we develop technology that produces radiation, and then simply look for means of increasing protection from radiation. Do you see this as being a satisfactory solution?

UPTON: First of all, we have no reason to think that there is a safe dose of radiation. There may be. It may turn out that tiny amounts of radiation are safe. But we suppose that even the smallest doses cause some risk.

The question then is, are the risks to which we expose ourselves acceptable ones? If I go to the dentist and he x-rays my teeth in efforts to prevent dental disease and the loss of my teeth, is that an acceptable risk? How do we decide?

We're now working very hard in radiological protection to quantify risks. When I got into this field, the debate raged as to whether there was a threshold. Many argued that small doses could be dismissed as essentially harmless. We don't argue that anymore. We want to measure the dose and estimate the risk. For me personally, if there were a better way to examine my teeth than using x-rays, I'd opt for it. But since there isn't, I accept the small dose — not because I know it's totally safe, but because it poses such a small risk to me as an individual, while affording such a potentially large benefit. I see this as an acceptable trade-off.

I know that if I go to Denver over the weekend, I'll get twice as much radiation as I will if I stay in New York City. But if I get an invitation to attend a meeting in the Rockies during the summer and get away from the heat and the humidity of the east coast, I go.

BRYANT: Does the increased radiation there have to do with the higher altitude?

UPTON: Yes. The effects of cosmic rays increase as we get closer to the top of the atmosphere. The earth is bombarded constantly from outer space with these rays.

BRYANT: There's not a higher incidence of cancer, though, in Colorado?

UPTON: Assuming that any amount of radiation causes some risk, we would predict an increased risk in Denver. However, when we look for a higher incidence of cancer there, we don't see it. This may be the result of a multitude of other variations from place to place.

BRYANT: What do you think is the most common stimulus for cancer formation in our environment?

UPTON: The most common stimulus for cancer formation in the environment is exposure to direct sunlight, and the most common cancer is cancer of the skin. About half of all skin cancer is related directly to sun exposure. I don't cover my head when I go out on a sunny day. I don't daub on sunblock. I have some lesions on my skin due to getting too much sun as a youth. But I accept the small risk of moderate dosages of sun for the pleasure of being out in the sunshine.

On the other hand, I wouldn't go to the beach on the first day of summer, lie out in the sun and get badly sunburned. That would make no sense.

BRYANT: Could you make a general statement as to the progress you've seen as a scientist working in the cancer field?

UPTON: We seem to have made almost miraculous progress since the 1940s in the treatment of childhood leukemia, Hodgkin's disease, choriocarcinoma, and juvenile soft-tissue tumors in general. Survival rates are vastly improved for those particular cancers.

On the other hand, I'm not aware of any really encouraging progress in treating many of the more common cancers—lung cancer, cancer of the pancreas, the colon, the breast—although some gains have been made in breast cancer.

BRYANT: Why do you feel that the cancer community as a whole has, historically, spent so much more time and money on the treatment of cancer rather than on the actual etiology of the disease?

UPTON: I think there are two reasons for this. One is that we tend, as human beings, to shoot the works to help our dear ones, our friends, our colleagues when they become ill and have need. We go to great ends and leave no stone unturned when it's our child, our parent, our sister or brother, husband or wife. We'd climb the highest mountain if we could save them or help them.

So we have every reason to pursue any approaches that look promising in terms of helping people who are already suffering. In general, I think, we spend very much less effort to prevent cancer because we haven't had a very good knowledge of the etiology of cancer as a biological phenomenon.

The prevention effort seems like a very long shot, usually. One is less prepared to spend large sums today for an uncertain, remote chance of benefits years in the future. To a certain extent, we can chalk this up to "human nature." There's something peculiar about us when it comes to prevention. Of course, some of us are more prevention-minded than others, but in general, we tend to opt for the cure.

BRYANT: We also tend to opt for ways which are consistent with our economic structure.

UPTON: Yes. One of the most cruel jokes, it seems to me, is the situation we have with smoking. I call it a joke, but it's anything but funny. We have good reason to think that there are perhaps one hundred thousand deaths in this country every year from cancer caused by smoking. One would think that society would turn itself inside out to exploit that information and to do what needs to be done to prevent those smoking-related cancer deaths. But, on the contrary, in our magazines, on our billboards, in our buses and taxis, we see a very vigorous, expensive, carefully contrived advertising campaign to promote smoking.

We see tax laws to protect the interests of the tobacco industry. We see flagrant mockery of the fact that this is a dreadful social problem that leads to a terrible disease. It's obvious that something could be done to prevent that toll of suffering.

BRYANT: Which makes it even more difficult to understand the American medical system's willingness to spend such vast amounts of money on treating the symptoms of cancer, rather than dealing primarily with the cause.

UPTON: Yes, I think that has been a weakness of American medicine. There has been, in my view, an overemphasis on diagnosis and treatment at the expense of etiology and prevention. Leadership from organized medicine has not been as strong as it could have been.

As director of the National Cancer Institute I struggled to assure myself and the American people that the program was properly balanced, and that we were utilizing our funds in a way that could be justified. I was, and am, concerned about what I see as a tendency to neglect cause and prevention in American medicine. So I struggled with the issue of spending; I tried to see to it that we were not neglecting cause and prevention in order to put increased funding into treatment.

BRYANT: You've been dealing with a great many ethical issues through the years. What do you see as being the most important ethical question related to cancer research and treatment today?

UPTON: It's hard for me to identify *the* most important question, though I can identify some of the important ones. One is
the "right to know" issue. We subscribe, as a society, to the belief
that people have a right to know about what might affect our lives.
If I know something which might affect your life, and I don't tell
you, then I'm denying you information which you have just as much
a right to know as I have.

This sounds reasonable to most of us who accept it as a valid
concept. But with cancer there's a problem, in that we're limited
in our ability to predict outcomes. If I examine your cells and discover that you have some chromosomal abnormalities, I might tell
you this and let you know that these abnormalities may be
manifestations of an injury that could predispose you to cancer.
And this might cause you some concern and worry. I don't know
what the risk is, though. It might conceivably be zero. The question then arises, should you tell someone — should you give someone information, the full significance of which you yourself can't
evaluate?

On the other hand, if I examine your blood and find that you've
been exposed to the virus associated with AIDS, my ethical responsibilities are clear. My not telling you would be a serious breach
of ethics and a threat to public health.

BRYANT: This seems closely related to the issue of a patient's
right to die.

UPTON: It is. Let's say I diagnose an advanced malignancy and
the statistics argue that the chance of cure is close to zero. If the
treatment is arduous, and if the patient is tired, sick, and doesn't
want to be treated, what are the rights of that patient? And how
do we support him in his struggle with the choice of submitting
to treatment or not? If the patient decides not to be treated, then
how do we help him to die with dignity and a minimum of
suffering?

The hospice approach has been generally accepted in this country. But though it looks simple on the surface, it involves, I'm sure
in every case, formidable ethical issues.

BRYANT: Can you relate this to the issue of cancer etiology?

UPTON: Sure. We have evidence that cancer often results from
man-made influences — whether or not we smoke, what we eat,
where we work, the chemicals and radiation levels we're exposed
to, and so on. We don't understand most of these influences pre-

cisely enough to know what the risks may be in a given situation yet, but we do have models. The very use of these models then leads to ethical questions. If a small amount of a material might kill people from cancer, shouldn't we then regulate exposure in order to protect people? By setting up or not setting up a body of standards, do we not then decide who is to live and who is to die?

BRYANT: That opens up the whole vista of industry and industrial products, and the role of the government's regulatory commissions.

UPTON: Exactly. Depending on how we set standards, whether it's for formaldehyde or benzene or something else, by regulating the amount of a given substance we allow workers to receive, we determine how many potential deaths there may be. Those are weighty ethical questions—balancing the rights and safety of individuals against the immediate convenience and economic well-being of society.

We must strive to achieve an acceptable balance between the uses of technology that enrich our lives and the misuses of technology that hurt people, including those people who will follow us in future generations. We have learned—painfully, over the past few years—that we are part of a fragile ecosystem. And we've learned that we can unwittingly damage this system, perhaps beyond repair. We can extinguish species unintentionally. With our nuclear weapons we may unintentionally extinguish the human race.

So it's imperative to understand what the implications of our technological developments may be for human safety in the years to come. This way, we may achieve a proper balance—beneficial, wholesome uses of technology, and the avoidance of technological abuses.

BRYANT: We have a tendency to go along blithely without recognizing the harm we may be inflicting on ourselves and on others.

UPTON: At least we're striving, in toxicology, to develop predictive techniques. We're using cellular models to help us identify potentially dangerous substances which could, fifty years from now, turn out to have caused cancer in many people. I see these as very auspicious and promising developments, but again, our knowledge is limited.

It gets back to the ethical question: do we, on the basis of one of these tests, ban a pesticide which might be very beneficial to farmers, or which might prevent malaria in certain populations?

Or ban a food additive that might preserve shelf life or even eliminate hunger in certain sectors? We face these questions constantly, and we desperately need socially acceptable answers which
involve ethical and technical judgments.

BRYANT: Of course, any decision that's made will involve economic factors as well.

UPTON: Precisely. If I spend money cleaning up the water, I may
not have money left to improve the playground. Is it better to have
kids on the street getting into mischief, getting run over, or is it
better to have clean water? Or can we strive for some of each, and
if so, how much of each?

These are the problems that one faces, requiring trade-offs based
on technological judgments and ethical considerations.

BRYANT: Once we recognize that some money-making product
is doing harm to our environment, how can we stop it? At what
point do we decide that the damage outweighs the benefits?

UPTON: That point is a moving target, I'm afraid. It rides with
the times. We went through a flush of concern and enthusiasm
for protecting the environment in the 1960s and early '70s. Rachel
Carson's book, *Silent Spring,* helped to raise public consciousness
of the specific nature of the problem. There was a great deal of
well-intentioned regulatory action, not all as deeply based in science
as it might have been. Meanwhile, during the '80s, we've experienced a reaction to all this—fear that we've gone too far, and
that regulations are strangling industry and private initiative. So
an effort is being made to back away to some extent.

However, legal precedents set during the '60s and '70s make it
very unlikely that we'll ever fully dismantle our regulatory establishment and go back to a laissez-faire situation.

I think we're going to live through a period of painful trial and
error, and adjustment. As we receive information about previously unforeseen risks, we'll try to deal with that information. We won't
know enough to adjust our regulations precisely; we may over-
regulate; we may under-regulate sometimes. It's going to take time,
as we improve our information and gain experience, to arrive at
fully justifiable and fully acceptable regulatory policies.

BRYANT: What is your long-range prognosis of the situation?

UPTON: I'm not a pessimist about the environment or the direction in which we're moving. I think, over the long haul, that things
are going to get better. Things *are* better. We're cleaning up toxic-
waste dumps. There are laws that protect the environment. They

may not be altogether enforced, but again, I think people are concerned. Nobody wants to live in a waste dump. Citizens' groups go snooping around, looking for signs of trouble. And scientists are doing ecological studies. Wherever there's a sniff of trouble, you're going to have a public outcry. Something will be done. That's healthy.

I think that what people need is enough information to keep things in perspective. Scientists on both sides of the issue exaggerate in one way or another, as do special-interest groups. The public is just going to have to learn to be a little bit suspicious and skeptical, and not believe everything it's told.

I'm optimistic about the future, basically. But I don't want to suggest that we're in the clear—that we know enough so that we'll never make any more mistakes or have any more arguments. We're going to go through a lot more grief before we get to that point.

BRYANT: What do you see as the most significant breakthrough in the cancer field during the past ten years or so?

UPTON: I think the most significant breakthrough in the last one or two decades has been the discovery of the oncogenes. We've known for a long time that inherited determinants affect susceptibility to cancer. We've produced cancer in animals by damaging chromosones and genes, using radiation or other chemotoxic materials.

As we begin to fish out the specific genes that appear to be activated in causing cancer, we come much closer to finding out about the disorder in cell regulation that causes the disease. I suspect we'll discover that there are dozens of such oncogenes, and that it's not just the oncogene itself which causes the cancer, but disturbance of the regulatory apparatus that normally functions to keep it in check. I think we're getting closer now to an understanding—an ability to define the chemical disturbance.

We are, all of us, chemical factories. And when things go wrong, they go wrong because the chemical reactions occur in the wrong sequence or to the wrong degree. Up until now we'd been groping to find out what these fundamental chemical reactions were. When we get there, we'll have an idea of what kinds of reactions go wrong. This will help us to recognize a problem in advance, before a tumor actually arises. Then we'll see what reactions are starting to go haywire. And perhaps we'll also have a way of correcting, through drugs or chemical modifiers, the faulty chemistry that makes the cancer cell what it is.

I'm very hopeful about this development, and I think it's a major breakthrough.

BRYANT: As chairman of the Institute of Environmental Medicine, do you have a message to share about something we may not have explored during this meeting?

UPTON: The first thing that comes to mind is the need to develop new energy technologies.

BRYANT: Safer energy sources?

UPTON: There is simply no safe form of electrical energy. Any form of electrical energy involves some hazards. Just transmitting electricity involves the danger of electrocution. We accept electric light bulbs because they are less dangerous than candles or gas. We accept nuclear power because, on the basis of all the studies that have been undertaken, the risks of nuclear power seem to be smaller than the risk of using coal.

If we had abundant supplies of natural gas, that would be better, but gas is running out, so we'll have to turn to other sources. Personally, I'd like to see us develop nuclear *fusion* energy because I think that would be a lot safer than nuclear fission, which we're involved with now. Fusion leaves no radioactive waste product.

Ultimately, though, I would like to see us learn to use the sun. I think we're certainly on the wrong track when we work on burning more and more biomass. That process just increases the carbon dioxide in the air. In fact, if we continue to burn fossil fuel or any carbonaceous material at present rates of consumption, we'll be contributing to massive, cataclysmic climate changes.

I hope society will do the research it needs to do in order to estimate risks as reliably as possible, and then try to make responsible decisions — choosing trade-offs that maximally protect future generations.

To me, burning up oil by driving big cars around is an obscene waste of resources. We're denying our grandchildren supplies of energy that are relatively cheap, plentiful and useful, just so we can enjoy a kind of luxury that to me is totally indefensible. Most people have not thought about this enough to be able to make carefully considered decisions. And we're being constantly manipulated by vested interests. Buy a big car. Put a tiger in your tank. Get four hundred fifty horsepower under the hood. Our descendants are going to resent that. They are not going to have that kind of fuel availability. Energy is going to be a lot more difficult to obtain. I hope that we will succeed at developing fusion power or abundant solar energy through direct electrical conversion.

BRYANT: Direct electrical conversion?

UPTON: Yes, using solar wafers like those used by space ships. The energy from the sun impinges on these cells and is converted directly into electrical energy. The wafers themselves actually absorb the sunlight. And in absorbing the sunlight, they produce electrical energy which is perfectly clean. It doesn't liberate effluents into the atmosphere: no carbon dioxide, no polyaromatic hydrocarbons, no waste.

A Macrobiotic Approach to Eating and Living

MICHIO KUSHI

*A leading figure in the international natural foods movement,
Michio Kushi is a philosopher, nutritional counselor and teacher. He
dedicated his early years to the study of international law at Tokyo
University, and after World War II became interested in world peace
through world government. Inspired by George Ohsawa, the father
of modern macrobiotics, who revised and introduced the principles
of Oriental philosophy and medicine to the West, Michio Kushi began a lifelong study of the application of traditional understanding
to solving problems of the modern world.*

*Michio Kushi is founder of the East West Foundation, which is
dedicated to the development of macrobiotic theory and practice; the
East West Journal, a monthly magazine which harmonizes traditional
Oriental philosophy, medicine and other aspects of culture with Western medical science; and Erewhon, a leading distributor of natural
and macrobiotic foods in North America. Actively working with other
organizations and individuals who share concerns such as health and
world peace, Michio Kushi has also inspired the founding of over three
hundred macrobiotic education centers throughout the Americas, Europe and the Far East. The Kushi Institute, founded to prepare macrobiotic instructors for their work, has branches in Boston, London,
Antwerp, Florence, Amsterdam and Bern.*

*Michio Kushi is the author of thirteen books, the most compre-
hensive of which are* The Cancer Prevention Diet *and* The Macrobiotic Way: The Complete Macrobiotic Diet and Exercise Book.
Others include The Book of Macrobiotics, Diet for a Strong Heart
and Macrobiotic Diet.

INTRODUCTION

I was first introduced to macrobiotics during the early 1970s. Living as an artist in Denmark, I spent a great deal of time at the Mu Club, a macrobiotic center based on the teachings of George Ohsawa (1893-1966). We were all experimenters, trying to understand and integrate the ancient tradition of macrobiotics with our modern Western conditioning and dietary habits of meat, potatoes, sweets and stimulants.

Daily, I read from George Ohsawa's "bible," *The Philosophy of Oriental Medicine.* I began to understand the principle of yin/yang, sky/earth, expansion/contraction; but like so many Westerners, my own tendency was to test the system by going to extremes. Although I don't recommend such an approach, fortunately for me, it served as an opening.

I saw results as I began to achieve a balance in my diet. I was able to recognize the qualities of yin and yang in the foods I ate, and became aware of how each quality affected my physical and psychological well-being. The deeper I explored, the greater became my sensitivity.

For many reasons, I have not followed a macrobiotic diet religiously since those early days in Copenhagen. But the basic principles of macrobiotics have very much affected my way of looking at food, and at the world. Macrobiotics has helped me to see that food, besides serving as nourishment, can also act as medicine, or poison. Through the years, I've come to believe that understanding and choosing the food we eat is as important as anything we shall ever do in this life. Surely, our eating habits contribute as much to our physical condition of health or sickness as do adequate fresh air, sunlight, exercise, and our ability to deal with stress. And food is one of the health factors that we can each control.

But macrobiotics is more than just a diet. Based on living in harmony with one's environment and the seasons, the philosophy behind macrobiotics supports ecological balance and world peace.

During the spring and summer of 1985 I had been studying Michio Kushi's book, *The Cancer Prevention Diet,* which includes macrobiotic theory, descriptions of various diseases, dietary recommendations, recipes and home remedies. As this work answered many questions I'd harbored for years, I wrote the author a letter requesting a meeting, and was honored to receive his gracious acceptance.

DIALOGUE

KUSHI: Balance is at the center of macrobiotic theory. Yin (expanding) and yang (contracting) energies interact as part of a cycle of eternal change. Attributes such as weight, temperature, shape, form, climate and culture can all be characterized as relatively yin or yang. Foods, too, range from extreme yang—animal products, processed salt—to extreme yin—refined foods, sugar and additives. The macrobiotic diet introduces the most highly balanced foods in relation to one's environment, in an attempt to strengthen the body's natural reserves and immune system. In temperate climates these foods include whole grains, locally grown vegetables in season, legumes, seaweed, and easily digested fermented products.

BRYANT: Although most Westerners think of macrobiotics as a new phenomenon, in your book, *The Cancer Prevention Diet,* you state that macrobiotics has been used by most of humankind for hundreds of generations to maintain health and resistance to disease, including cancer. Can you explain?

KUSHI: The macrobiotic way of eating is a widespread, traditional way of nourishment, which has been practiced for as long as people have lived on this planet. Macrobiotics is based upon our harmonious relationship with the natural environment. It involves eating the whole foods that grow around us.

In temperate climates, whole grains have always been cultivated as a staple food. Fresh vegetables were prepared in various ways as a secondary food. Protein naturally came mostly from vegetable sources. Fruits were eaten *in season.* In coastal locations, seaweed has always been eaten as a valuable mineral supplement.

Organic grains, vegetables and beans have formed the backbone of most traditional diets for thousands of years. This way of eating transcends the differences between cultures, races and religions. Macrobiotic principles are based on the simple human practices of living in harmony with nature.

BRYANT: During the last three generations or so, since modern technologies were applied to what has become the "food industry," we've seen a great many changes.

KUSHI: Yes, both in the food itself, and in people's eating patterns. Chemicalization, refinement, mass production, and food processing have compromised the quality of the food we eat, while modern agricultural practices and our demand for foods grown in other climates contribute further to the lowering of our natural immunitites.

Our modern diet emphasizes fatty foods, including dairy products and meat, while de-emphasizing the importance of whole grains and vegetables. I make a correlation between this trend and the fact that cancer and other degenerative diseases are on the rapid increase today.

In Japan, when I was young, cancer was very rare. Even in 1949, when I arrived in America, cancer threatened just one out of every seven people. Now it threatens one out of three.

BRYANT: But isn't this greatly due to environmental problems which have become more serious since World War II?

KUSHI: To some extent, this increase is due to our creation of various environmental problems, such as water and air pollution. But there have always been environmental problems to face in every culture, in every age. In traditional cultures, where people ate and lived in accordance with the basic macrobiotic principles, changes in environmental quality could be withstood much better, because the macrobiotic way of eating helps to build resistance to illness through the development of natural adaptation to the environment. In this way it can prevent cancer and other degenerative diseases.

BRYANT: You've mentioned that one of the basic principles of macrobiotics is living in harmony with nature. But in the twentieth century, it's hard for some of us to visualize what is meant by that. Can you go into some detail about what this sort of living entails?

KUSHI: In terms of diet, it means that we eat according to the geography and climate of our immediate environment. When the season changes, we naturally change our cooking style. Being in harmony with nature also means that if we are living in New England, we should not depend on foods which come from a tropical climate, nor should we depend on foods which have been chemically processed.

Buckwheat, rice, wheat, barley, millet, and other grains compose fifty to sixty percent of a natural diet in four-season areas of the world. In contrast, the traditional diet of cold, polar regions consists mostly of animal food, as has been practiced for many centuries. In a very hot climate, we will find the people depending more upon subtropical and tropical products, and practicing very different means of preparing food in accordance with the climate and the resources available. Nothing could be more ancient, or more logical.

BRYANT: Certainly the radiation we're all exposed to in our environment—from the sun, televisions and computers, x-rays, microwaves, and other common sources—is a great contributor to cancer. But I understand that in Japan, some residents of areas contaminated with radiation from the atomic bomb of 1945 followed the macrobiotic program, and were able to offset the effects of radiation. It's surprising that anything so simple as diet can be so effective against threats as serious as radiation. Can you talk about how the macrobiotic diet does this?

KUSHI: When Nagasaki received the atomic bomb, St. Francis Hospital was located in the central region of the explosion. Dr. Akizuki, the hospital director, followed a macrobiotic program. He encouraged his entire staff and all of the hospital's patients to practice macrobiotics. After the bomb hit, they ate brown rice and seaweed, miso soup, winter squash, other cooked vegetables, and sea salt. And although they had to wait several days for help to come from outside, those people were safe, while many surrounding people were dead.

Studies have shown that the brown part of whole grains contains a certain acid which can chemically unite with and discharge radioactive factors such as Strontium-90. Minerals contained in seaweed have the same kind of effect, as do various wild grasses when properly prepared. So does miso. Scientific studies have revealed that people who eat the macrobiotic way can eliminate the effects of radiation.

People who eat dairy food, sugars and meat show far greater effects of radiation: more burning, more spreading of the radiation throughout the body. Of course, in the case of extremely high doses of radiation, food would not make nearly as much difference. But in cases of so-called moderate exposure, the macrobiotic way of eating is extremely advantageous.

BRYANT: As you know, Ann Wigmore is also committed to the nutritional approach to preventing and curing disease. But you have great differences. How do the principles she works with compare with yours?

KUSHI: It's interesting that Ann Wigmore named her program after Hippocrates. The essence of his teaching was to approach disease through changes in diet, environment, and other aspects of one's lifestyle. Medical application was administered sparingly. His advice was, "If you try to deal with illness using drastic means,

you'll die sooner. If you just change your diet and lifestyle, you'll
live much longer."

Hippocrates actually called his approach "macro-biotics," and his
views are entirely compatible with modern macrobiotics. His views
were shared by many pre-Socratic thinkers and healers such as
Aristotle and Galen.

Let's look at why they called their food "living food." If we put
a grain of whole rice into the ground, it will grow, even one hundred years from now. It is alive. But refined grains cannot grow.
The life-giving principle has been removed.

We use living foods in macrobiotics—whole foods: the greens
of carrots, beets, turnips, as well as the roots. We use whole beans:
aduki beans, chick peas, lentils, all with the capacity for sprouting
and growing. All of these are living foods. We don't use refined or
processed foods. No canned vegetables. Our idea and Hippocrates'
idea are in total accord.

However, Ms. Wigmore has taken this "living foods" principle
to the extreme of eating only raw foods. I think this certainly has
its value as a temporary measure in order to detoxify the body of
animal food. Wheat grass can help the body to eliminate toxins,
and can be quite useful in an acute situation for someone who
has eaten eggs, meat, greasy foods and dairy foods over a long period
of time.

BRYANT: For how long would you recommend a person to maintain the Hippocrates Living Foods diet?

KUSHI: A detoxification could take anywhere from one week to
three months.

For a person who has been a vegetarian for a while, this diet
would not be very helpful. It's not in harmony with the seasons
to eat tropical foods in cold weather, for instance.

It doesn't help the body to maintain a balance. Someone with
a very strong constitution, like Anne Wigmore herself, can take
the raw Living Foods diet for an extended period. Someone with
a more fragile constitution would certainly weaken on that diet
over a long period of time.

BRYANT: Do you feel that "living foods" can be successfully integrated with macrobiotics in helping people to make a transition
between a heavy meat, dairy and refined-foods diet to a more
balanced one?

KUSHI: Certainly, in transitional cases. In less acute conditions,
I recommend a gradual approach to macrobiotics. A person may

eat less meat, dairy products, fats, sugars and refined foods and eat more whole grains, fish and vegetables. In general I think a gradual approach is the most sound.

BRYANT: There's room then, for varied approaches to diet as a means of improving general health.

KUSHI: No group should claim that its way is the only way—especially when they aren't able to keep themselves from getting the very diseases they're treating. I would like to see cancer doctors free of cancer and heart doctors free of heart disease. But instead of focusing primarily on their own health and the health of their communities, many health professionals are focusing their energy on creating a monopoly of control over medicine. This is an extension of the same dualism which pits people of different races, religions and political ideas against each other as opponents.

The general public pays for medical care. The people who pay for this service are the employers, so they should be able to explore medical treatments of every stripe. This is a basic freedom. It's a grave error when patients forget that they are the employers and act as if they were subjects of the health professionals. It contributes to a narrow view of medicine and a narrow view of health.

BRYANT: Many people today are experiencing various symptoms of unbalanced health without being able to figure out what's wrong. Can you describe some precancerous symptoms as a means of helping people to become aware that it may be time to effect some changes?

KUSHI: People who have allergies, sinus congestion, vaginal discharge, and greasy skin ruptures, are experiencing pre-cancerous conditions. If they continue to eat low quality food excessively, cancer will set in, five, ten or twenty years later.

Different cancers are caused by different habits. For instance, colon and prostate cancer originate in a diet heavy with meat consumption. Others, such as breast cancer, result from excessive intake of dairy food, ice cream, and sugars combined with poultry, meat and other oily, greasy foods.

It's important that people realize that cancer is not some independent condition. Cancer is caused by unhealthy eating and living over time. Before cancer appears, many symptoms appear. Sometimes it may take the form of fatigue, sometimes mucus discharge, etc. People don't notice, and think these are independent problems that can be named and treated according to their symptoms. People then treat the symptoms, which they see as unrelated, and so they forget that the next health problem is related to the first. They ignore the progression of their illness.

By the time an illness manifests as cancer, the symptoms are rather dramatic. The person may notice fat accumulation or weight loss and increased tension. Cysts may form, the skin may rupture. These are all signs of cancer.

BRYANT: Can you talk about some of the diagnostic principles and techniques you've adapted from the East as part of the modern macrobiotic program?

KUSHI: Traditionally, we use many ways of evaluating our health. We can use visual means. We can analyze one's pulse. We can listen carefully to a patient's words and means of self-expression. We can observe the patient's activities or physical movements. We can observe the patient's living conditions and general environment. We analyze the patient's diet. We become aware of a personal vibration, which some may call an "aura." And we probe certain pressure points of the body to find sensitive areas. When people become aware of these diagnostic tools, they can help themselves a great deal.

Many cancers can be detected by observation of the skin alone. A greenish hue may denote cancer. For instance, a cancer of the large intestine may show itself as a greenish hue between the thumb and first finger. The small intestine meridian is located on the side of the hand near the little finger. This is a general concept. If the greenish hue appears along the wrist, we are shown a cancer of an upper area of the body, like lungs or breasts. Along the outside of the foot, a green color means that the reproductive organs are in trouble. If the green hue appears on the inside of the foot and up the leg, we see evidence of spleen or liver-related cancer.

BRYANT: How does being overweight affect the likelihood of one getting cancer?

KUSHI: Fatty accumulation tends to inhibit energy circulation. The result is stagnation. Fatty deposits, cysts, even tumors can then be formed. Excessive dairy-food consumption is dangerous for this reason. It helps to form fatty layers underneath the skin.

BRYANT: When you change from a diet characterized by meat and dairy products to a macrobiotic diet, how long does it take before the body is free of the effects of previous eating patterns?

KUSHI: It takes the body several years to get rid of all animal byproducts, but within six months to one year, many changes will have taken place, and the person is much, much safer.

BRYANT: How long does it take to rid the body of the effects of most drugs?

KUSHI: It depends on the volume and the kind of drug used. If once in a blue moon someone smokes marijuana, it may take just two weeks to rid the system of it. But it might take a habitual smoker much longer. Stronger drugs take a longer time — from two to seven years.

BRYANT: What about cigarettes?

KUSHI: It takes about two to three years to be completely free of the effects of cigarettes smoked over a long period of time, but after just two months, most effects are gone.

BRYANT: In *The Cancer Prevention Diet*, you say that cancer results from the body's healthy attempt to isolate toxins ingested and accumulated through years of eating a modern, unnatural diet and living in an artificial environment. Could you elaborate on this?

KUSHI: Normally, we discharge wastes through urination, bowel movement, perspiration, coughing, sneezes and fevers. But if we keep eating dairy products, refined foods and chemicalized foods, our eliminative functions become weakened and our kidneys are unable to discharge smoothly. As a result, chronic accumulation begins.

The body continues to function through all of this difficulty. It may accumulate discharge in one area of the body in order to save the entire organism. Tumors actually help the body to avoid contracting generalized and fatally toxic conditions. The whole body would be poisoned if we didn't create individualized cancers. If one continues to eat excessive amounts of dairy and other undesirable fatty food, a localized tumor may grow bigger, blocking important body functions; or another tumor may be created. If a cancer patient has surgery, yet still continues to eat the same foods, the tumor will find another place in which to develop.

BRYANT: What about women who undergo operations to remove part of their breasts in order to prevent breast cancer?

KUSHI: It's ridiculous. Such surgery is like removing one's tonsils, which are part of our lymphatic system. When we eat sugar and dairy products, infected tonsils warn us that we're creating a toxic condition. Without our tonsils, we lose some of our natural immunity.

BRYANT: These days, our natural immune systems are being seriously threatened. I'm thinking especially of the widespread occurrence of AIDS. What do you see as being the cause of this?

KUSHI: No matter what the catalyst, AIDS is the product of an exhausted immune system. Many AIDS patients have taken drugs, ranging from antibiotics to marijuana, over a long period of time. Plus, as modern Westerners, they've weakened their systems through habitual consumption of sugars, sweets and greasy foods, which have also contributed to a condition of chronic mineral depletion.

We're doing a great deal of research on macrobiotics and AIDS. Of course, much more research is needed, but we find that macrobiotic AIDS patients are sustaining their health, and some of them are improving.

BRYANT: Can you explain the process the body goes through when one with a serious disease goes on the macrobiotic diet?

KUSHI: Many cancer patients start to feel that their digestive systems function much better and that their mental abilities improve. Physical energy is restored. All this happens within one month. Also, if one is overweight, one will start to lose weight; if too thin, one will start to gain weight. Some people may experience skin problems, vaginal discharge or coughing, as accumulated fat starts to discharge. And as time goes by, they become sounder sleepers; verbal expression becomes clearer; they have more energy, and the cancer symptoms themselves, including pain, often begin to disappear. Of course, this depends upon the severity of the condition and proper maintenance of the program.

In the beginning, some people may feel that the cancer itself is growing, while the whole body seems to be improving. That's because as the body cleans itself out, toxins may be stored in a localized place such as the tumor site. Within six months' time, though, the cancer frequently starts to recede.

BRYANT: Do you see macrobiotics as being effective when used in conjunction with cancer treatments such as chemotherapy, radiation or surgery?

KUSHI: Some patients combine chemotherapy, radiation or surgery with macrobiotics. In treating their condition in this way, the macrobiotic diet itself must be modified. For instance, chemotherapy affects protein and fat absorption. So a carefully balanced macrobiotic diet would include more sources of protein and fat, such as fish and oils. More sweets, such as barley malt, may be employed in such a case, because chemotherapy also causes a craving for sweets. Cooked fruits could then supplement the usual grains, soup, legumes and vegetables. Radiation calls for increased consumption of miso soup and seaweed, which are taken along with whole grains and vegetables.

However, the most important consideration in such cases is the cooperation and support of the patient's family and physician. The physician must understand that the macrobiotic approach is not harmful, and that it can complement whatever medical procedure is being used.

BRYANT: The patient's family could play an important supportive role here. Cooking and eating habits are hard to break, and it's almost impossible when those around us are enjoying modern refined foods, sweets, dairy products, and other nontraditional forms of nourishment.

KUSHI: That's true. It's very important for the family to eat together as frequently as possible. In fact, in *every* case I know of in which a terminal cancer patient has survived using macrobiotics and standard therapy, the patient had the full support of his or her family. When a woman is suffering from cancer, and her husband says, "Cook for yourself. I want steak, not vegetables," the situation is probably hopeless.

BRYANT: Such a lack of understanding and support within a household could even have helped to cause a person's illness to begin with.

KUSHI: Exactly. Family problems and tensions can always contribute to illness.

BRYANT: Along with diet and a caring environment, what do you recommend for people as part of a complete macrobiotic approach?

KUSHI: The macrobiotic approach includes the practice of light, comfortable, physical exercise. Herbal medicines may also be administered along with acupuncture or acupressure. And extremely important is the cultivation of a relaxed, peaceful mind. Meditation is very helpful.

BRYANT: From what you say, I gather that environment, activities, and attitude all play a part in a person's ability to work with macrobiotics successfully. Yet the most important factor seems to be the food we eat and how it is prepared.

KUSHI: I cannot emphasize enough how important cooking is — how important it is to be able to use all that cooking knowledge that our grandmothers and great-grandmothers practiced.

BRYANT: It almost sounds as if you're saying that the way we cook our food is as important as the food itself.

KUSHI: Cooking is energizing! And we give our food different types of energies depending upon the methods we choose: applying fire, applying pressure, drying, steaming, salt treatment, soup-making, fermenting, pickling. Each of these methods has its own special effect on the way food is utilized by the body. When combined with a relaxed, peaceful mind, and a sense of caring and love for the people being fed, cooking becomes the highest art.

BRYANT: I imagine that the practice of macrobiotics on a large scale has the capacity to greatly affect society. For instance, eating that which is grown in one's geographical location has economic and even political ramifications.

KUSHI: The macrobiotic diet is a part of something much greater. Macrobiotics is part of an understanding about the universe, and about what life is. Macrobiotic living is the practice of common, basic, human values applied not only to food, but to spiritual, mental and physical practices. Macrobiotics leads to peaceful, harmonious relations with other peoples and societies, and respect for cultural traditions. Macrobiotics teaches cooperation with nature, and supports one's ability to marvel at and appreciate nature. So the social and political implications of eating traditional, whole foods are very great.

First of all, macrobiotics minimizes the occurrence of degenerative diseases. This saves billions of health care dollars each year. I have no objection to the medical establishment's growth, or to making various kinds of medical care available, but presently, many people are almost totally dependent on health care professionals, forgetting about their own responsibility and their own healing capabilities. For instance, it's very important to see how our day-to-day eating habits and living habits can either keep us healthy and strong or cause various types of sickness.

BRYANT: What about mental illness? Do you have any evidence of the effect of a macrobiotic diet on mental health?

KUSHI: Yes. It has been shown that people who eat macrobiotically experience very little mental imbalance, and perpetrate far fewer crimes. Of course, mental illness and crime have a tremendous impact on society. So the work of macrobiotics is the work of making the world as a whole much more peaceful and harmonious.

BRYANT: Do you feel that changes in diet adopted on a large scale will affect our chances for world peace?

KUSHI: Yes, definitely. There is a connection between the kind of society we live in and the high-protein, high-fat, chemicalized foods we eat. This sort of eating can produce a wide range of symptoms, from depression to hypertension and nervous disorders. One's disposition and response to stimuli are greatly dependent upon the food one has been eating over many years' time. And these qualities can be modified through dietary changes.

The biological, biochemical changes which come through proper diet and living in harmony with nature will allow us to accept the differences of others, while ridding ourselves of unnecessary aggression. This state of being will allow us to develop a healthy, peaceful standard.

Today all mankind faces the threat of nuclear disaster, but what is really the cause of war? There are many theories about war's cause. People blame imperialism, racism, economics. But all these things have their roots in a much more basic cause. War is very much a biological or biopsychological problem. And it is of utmost importance that we understand the biological and biochemical status which will help us work toward peace in this world.

The macrobiotic principle contributes to a world vision which accepts cultural differences and embraces the traditional ways of all people. Through this understanding we may create a planetary constitution of humankind for the health and betterment of all, through the free will of all.

BRYANT: It's hard to imagine a truly unified planet in this age of aggressive international politics. What do you see as the motivating factor that will help the people and nations of the world to live in harmony?

KUSHI: The common motivation will be our individual health, first. This is the most immediate crisis. The next consideration is family health and happiness. Finally, our desire for the well-being of society and the world may unite us.

Fortunately for the future of the world, the social problems we face today force us to reflect upon the direction we've taken as a society. Our fears will help us to move toward finding solutions. We're seriously evaluating our progress and imagining ways of living which would be more conducive to physical, psychological and political health.

BRYANT: We are involved with a technological and social revolution which may or may not help us reach that state of health.

KUSHI: The purely mechanical approach to science tends to trivialize traditional values and ways of life. Medically speaking, we choose to control illnesses using drugs and electronic means. Without truly understanding the causes of disease, we remove parts of the body, mechanically stimulate our organs, and gradually artificialize our bodies. On the psychological level, we only understand the mechanical behaviors: if I give this chemical treatment, the patient will react this way. But what are the effects of such treatment? How is this treatment affecting the energy of the entire person? This we do not know.

In my view, we are now at a turning point in history. We may decide to go further on the road to the mechanization and artificialization of the human species, or we may decide to start turning toward more natural ways of living and caring for ourselves. *This is the point of decision.*

BRYANT: If macrobiotic theory could be applied to a system of technological development, how would that technology be characterized?

KUSHI: Today we are using limited natural resources as if they had no limit. We ignore the fact that using these resources has serious side effects in the form of pollution, and we ignore the possibility of developing technology which uses limitless universal energies. Why not learn to use the force that keeps this Earth rotating, the force that keeps the solar system intact and moving? Why not learn to use the energies which we receive constantly from the universe? These energies are helping our entire planet and even our entire solar system to work. Why don't we explore these methods? This is surely an important key to our advancement.

I think it is interesting that while we are worried about finding enough energy to move our cars, there are forces great enough to move the entire Earth. The entire Earth is moving! Certainly, we have access to the energy that moves the Earth. This is something we should explore.

The Work of a Biochemist-Physician

EMANUEL REVICI, M.D.

Dr. Emanuel Revici has been active since 1921 as an independent research scientist and physician. Although he is associated primarily with cancer therapy, his discoveries in the fields of microbiology, radiology, and biochemistry are applicable to a wide range of pathological conditions, including drug addiction, hemorrhage, rheumatoid arthritis, allergies, shock, impaired hearing, burns and arteriosclerosis.

Through his research, Emanuel Revici has observed that all natural systems involve the activity of two opposing processes: one destructive, and one constructive. The destructive or catabolic process moves rapidly toward entropy, the breakdown of structure. The anabolic process moves toward the growth and build-up of natural patterns. According to Dr. Revici, health is the maintenance of a dynamic balance between these two types of activity. A predominance of either catabolic or anabolic forces is the origin of abnormality, pain and disease. His non-toxic therapies are administered according to each individual's metabolic character and condition, which is determined by urine analysis and other tests.

Although Dr. Revici's approach to medicine is grounded in the traditional allopathic system, he has used his extensive training and laboratory experience to break ground in previously unexplored areas of scientific research and medical practice. His work in the field of biochemistry includes a practical theory about the organization of the periodic table. Einstein's Quantum Theory of Physics is fundamental to Dr. Revici's perspective.

The Institute of Applied Biology, Research and Activity Through 1983, a succinct introductory booklet describing Dr. Revici's in-

*terests and achievements, is available through the Institute of Ap-
plied Biology in New York City. Doctor Revici's major work, Research
in Physiopathology as Basis of Guided Chemotherapy with Special Application to Cancer, published for the American Foundation
for Cancer Research in 1961 by D. Van Nostrand, New York (772
pages) has been translated into German, and is currently being translated into Italian.*

*Originally from Rumania, Dr. Emanuel Revici made a small for-
tune as a research scientist when, during his early twenties, he developed and patented an oil-refining process which changed crude,
low-viscosity petroleum into valuable, high-grade oil needed by the
Rumanian aviation industry. During the 1930s, he was chief of the
laboratory of bacteriology at Bucharest's Faculty of Medicine, and highly respected by the European scientific community. He was welcomed
at laboratories and hospitals in Vienna, Paris, Berlin, Rome and London, where he studied, conducted research, and wrote about his
findings. By 1936, he had organized his own research teams and laboratories in France with the help of his oil patent royalties. He worked
there steadily until, having joined the French Resistance, he was forced
to flee from the Nazis in 1941. He then set up research laboratories,
first in Mexico and later in the U.S. Since 1947, his medical practice
(he directed Trafalgar Hospital until 1972) and laboratory, the Institute of Applied Biology, have been located in New York City.*

*While most of the mainstream work in immunology and im-
munotherapy has been directed toward proteins such as antibodies
and enzymes, Dr. Revici has focused more than sixty years of study
on the lipidic immune system. His research is based on the composition and polarized functions of fatty acids on one side, and sterols
on the other. Cancer, Revici has discovered, is promoted by substances
characterized by a sterolic (anabolic) molecular structure. Cholester-
ol is an example of an anabolic sterol; most carcinogens share anabolic activity. According to Revici, radiation, which creates the
abnormal fatty acids mentioned above, has a catabolic effect, which
in turn stimulates an anabolic defense reaction that in itself can promote cancer.*

*In treating disease, Dr. Revici first determines whether the cata-
bolic or anabolic phase of activity predominates. His treatment begins with a determination as to which phase is currently progressing
unchecked. Then lipid-based compounds, which have the capacity
of normalizing the relationship between anabolic and catabolic forces,
are administered carefully, in accordance with each patient's metabolic character. These medicines are changed as the patient's*

biochemical balance changes.

Through his approach, based upon but not limited to standard allopathic practice, Dr. Revici claims to work with a patient's individual chemical makeup. He explained recently, "We are strongly individualized, and strongly individualized are our diseases. In everybody, there are millions of genes, which combine to make biological, physiochemical, physiological, and pathological 'personalities.' There are simply no two cancers which are alike, just as no two individuals are alike."

INTRODUCTION

Dr. Revici's goal is, very simply, to help his fellow human beings, and he works tirelessly to attain this goal. Since our first meeting, I've spent several Sunday afternoons in his living room, amidst
tropical plants, microscopes, manuscripts piled from floor to ceil-
ing, and mementos from patients including theater celebrities, cabi-
net ministers, writers and ambassadors. During my visits, as I
document countless hours of discussion on audio and videotape,
he is constantly interrupted by calls from patients. It's clear that
he puts sixty-five years of medical experience to work as he listens
to them and recommends specific adjustments to therapy in response to metabolic changes.

Dr. Revici's treatments have proven extremely helpful to me in
treating long-term, lingering health problems which had stumped
various other doctors. And over the course of time, I've seen some
patients diagnosed with hopeless diseases experience remissions
and cures under his care.

On a personal level, his most memorable quality is his compassion and his genuine caring. On the level of science, his innovative work has faced resistance from the established medical
community. I look forward to the day when he is recognized for
his work in the field of biochemistry, and for his tremendous contributions to medicine.

DIALOGUE

NEW PERSPECTIVES

BRYANT: I understand that you've developed a description of cancer formation as it evolves from the precellular level to the levels of the cell and the tissue, and finally, as it affects the entire organism. It seems to me that this information could be of great value in helping to recognize and treat cancer before it actually attacks the organism as a full-blown, malignant condition. Can you talk about your discoveries?

REVICI: The basic idea is that cancer is initiated at the simplest level of biological organization as a manifestation of anabolic imbalance; that is, imbalance characterized by excessive growth or build up. Such imbalance, beginning at the molecular level of our makeup, may develop unchecked, eventually affecting more highly organized levels of the body.

We could call changes caused by such imbalance at the chromosomal stage, "pre-cancer." This happens long before individual cells, tissues or organs of the body are affected.

A partially developed form of cancer (noninvasive cancer or cancer-in-situ) is characterized by changes in the nuclei, though not yet in the cytoplasm of cells. At this stage, the cellular cytoplasm appears normal, but there are organizational abnormalities.

The next stage, malignancy, does not occur until the cells change further. Malignant cells are anabolic and invasive. They also take on other characteristics which do not exist in either the pre-cancer or the cancer-in-situ stages. Of course the invasive or malignant cells destroy healthy cells.

BRYANT: So, according to your findings, it would be a productive move for science to address itself not only to cancer in its malignant aspect, but also to the process of transformation from the state of pre-cancer to cancer-in-situ and invasive cancer.

REVICI: Yes. What's needed is an anticarcinogenic agent which would prohibit the passage of a precancerous condition to the stage of invasive or malignant cancer. According to our observations, the key to this development is linked with the body's lipidic system of defense. We at the Institute of Applied Biology have found that this defense system can be normalized when certain elements are introduced in the form of lipidic, fatty compounds.

BRYANT: You also use selenium compounds in treating cancer. Can you talk about that?

REVICI: Research has shown that people living near selenium-rich soil, eating selenium-rich food, experience a very low incidence of cancer. So, although other substances may be far more effective in the treatment of cancer, there is a great deal to be learned about selenium.

BRYANT: The U.S. government recommends a limit on selenium intake. Why?

REVICI: Too much selenite—hexavalent-positive selenium— has toxic effects on animals. So The National Academy of Science has limited the intake of hexavalent-positive selenium to a dosage of no more than one hundred or one hundred fifty micrograms by mouth. However, there are astonishing differences between the different forms of selenium. For instance, I use a bivalent-negative form of selenium, incorporated in a molecule of a fatty acid. This is such a different substance that I can administer up to one gram of selenium per day by injection (which is usually considered to be four times as powerful as what is administered by mouth). That corresponds to *one million* micrograms per day, and there are no toxic effects.

BRYANT: Have you found uses for selenium besides cancer prevention?

REVICI: Yes. We first utilized these high dosages of selenium in treating heroin addiction in more than two thousand patients. There were absolutely no toxic effects. The explanation for our success, and for the lack of toxicity, was the fact that I introduced the selenium inside a molecule of lipidic substance.

BRYANT: What kind of experiments have you done in order to find other cancer-prevention agents?

REVICI: I have found an entire series of agents which prevents the appearance of cancer in strains of animals, and in conditions under which a high proportion of cancer ordinarily appears.

Working with mice, we've found that, in general, the administration of anabolic agents—sterols, alcohols and amines, for instance—increases the percentage of spontaneous cancer, indicating very probably an action on the lower levels of biological organization. In general, catabolic substances reduce the percentage of spontaneous cancers.

BRYANT: Could you name the actual substances you're working with?

REVICI: Sodium thiosulfate, a catabolic compound, given the entire year by mouth in drinking water, had reduced the incidence of cancer in one experimental group from forty-seven percent to two percent. We investigated the toxicity of this substance, examining the mortality rate of one hundred animals. Our unexpected discovery was that not only did we have a smaller number of cancers in the group taking sodium thiosulfate, but we also observed a lower rate of mortality.

Mixing the substances, alternating injections of sodium thiosulfate with selenium, we obtained practically no spontaneous cancer. Neither substance has resulted in increased mortality in animals.

Another substance we've used successfully is called bixine, an acid obtained from the seeds of the plant, *Bixa orellana.* We used this very successfully, and continue to use it today in the treatment of cancer. We've also had good results with a form of fluorine.

BRYANT: I've read that fluorine actually has a light carcinogenic effect.

REVICI: Yes, but at the Institute, we've developed another form of fluorine. Like sulfur, selenium and bixine, it is effective as an anticarcinogen in certain circumstances.

We've also used parinaric acid, a highly unsaturated, tetra-enic conjugated fatty acid, obtained through the extraction of oils from the plant *Parinarium laurenum.* Interestingly, parinaric acid, characterized by four conjugated, double bonds, has a special action on carcinogens, practically annihilating the carcinogenic action or capacity of a substance.

Further experiments in this direction would certainly prove interesting. In the case of sulfur, for instance, we know that in order to have an anticarcinogenic property, sulfur must be bivalent-negative. Hexa- and tetravalent-positive forms of sulfur aren't active. The best results are with the bivalent-negative forms of sulfur combined with certain salts, or even bound with lipids. As I've mentioned, sodium thiosulfate offers a very high percentage of cancer prevention.

BRYANT: Have you worked with the various compounds you're describing in the context of human treatment, or only on the level of animal experimentation?

REVICI: It is practically impossible to recognize when cancer is actually being prevented in human beings. The only way to establish the proper experimental conditions would be to formulate something such as that which I proposed in China when I was invited there to give a series of lectures. In a place like China, it would be possible to take one half of an entire town and to give those people, every Sunday for instance, one of these cancer-preventive substances. The other half would refrain from taking these substances. After a determined amount of time, we would compare the proportion of cancer incidence in one half of the town with the other half. This is the only way to test a substance for activity in preventing cancer in humans. I would give selenium to one group; other groups would be given the other agents I've mentioned.

BRYANT: I know you are working with genetics. Are there ways of applying your findings in that field to pathological conditions like cancer?

REVICI: Yes. I've shown that the chemical constituents of genes are involved in activities which have never before been associated with those genes.

I began working with genes when I first studied the basic hierarchical development of biological entities. I think that my work may bring us to a better understanding of genetics.

For instance, with animals I've seen unbelievable results using genetic derivatives as therapeutic agents. Seriously ill animals with various conditions — animals who according to all evidence should have died within only hours — are still alive months later after being injected with certain substances obtained from animal genes.

BRYANT: You've had some success working with AIDS patients. Can you talk about your approach to treatment?

REVICI: The AIDS research I've been doing since 1980 is really an extension of work I began in 1939 when I became totally incapacitated following an experiment with a virus I hoped would help fight cancer. I was in an iron lung for months, thanks to the virus, so when I became well, I got totally involved in viral research.

For treatment of AIDS, which is caused by a virus, my plan involves three treatments: one is designed to inactivate or kill the virus itself; the other works to correct abnormalities within the lipidic defense system; third, medications are given to treat whatever added, opportunistic disease the body is currently facing due to a lack of immune response.

ON PAIN

BRYANT: I think that in most cultures it is agreed that part of our work as human beings is to help alleviate pain and suffering. From previous discussions with you, I know that your research on pain has led to some of your most important discoveries, including your discovery of the dualistic — catabolic/anabolic — metabolic process. Would you describe the evolution of this work?

REVICI: I began studying pathological pain, the pain of internally-caused abnormality and disease, in Paris during the 1930s as an independent research scientist. Working closely with over thirty terminal cancer patients, I observed some patients complaining that their pain increased during the morning, and that in the evening they felt much better. This happened also to be true in the case of my wife, who suffered from terrible headaches. In the morning, she was really sick from the pain, but in the evening she never felt pain at all. In fact, she could live in the evening as if she were perfectly well. Then in the morning she was barely able to lift her head from the pillow with the intensity of her pain.

At the same time, another group of patients claimed to feel much better in the morning. For them it was the evening which brought pain. This was very interesting to me.

BRYANT: How did you go about investigating this?

REVICI: I asked cancer patients who were in pain when their pain was the greatest. Interestingly, there were two sets of responses. One group experienced the severest pain only in the morning, while for the other group, it was only in the evening. *Not one person claimed that there was no difference.* It became clear to me that a kind of dualism was involved here.

BRYANT: Did you find that diet is in any way related to the pain or to the dualism itself?

REVICI: Only in a very general way. Morning pain is relieved by eating, while evening pain is exaggerated by eating. When I understood this, I felt I had hit upon some important correlations among food, pain and the time of day.

I already knew that the body's acid and alkaline balance changes throughout the day, in most cases becoming more alkaline toward evening. I also knew that immediately after eating, the body becomes strongly alkalinized. This phenomenon is called an "alkaline tide."

BRYANT: For those of us with a less scientific orientation, can you describe the alkaline tide in a little more detail?

REVICI: The alkaline tide occurs because during digestion hydrochloric acid enters the stomach. The chloride ions come from sodium chloride, and the remaining free sodium ions bond with free carbonates to form alkaline substances such as sodium bicarbonate. The result is that a state of alkalinity exists for ten to twenty minutes after eating, until the sodium is secreted in the duodenum, where it once again bonds the chlorides that come from the stomach to form sodium chloride—salt—which can be absorbed entirely.

With this awareness of alkaline tide, it now became clearer to me how the acid/alkaline balance of the body is related to both eating and the time of day. I saw a connection between the intensity of morning and evening pain and the acid/base condition of the body caused by time of day or by food ingestion. It was now a question only of showing a correlation between the acid/base balance of the body and the dualism of pain.

BRYANT: I'm familiar with the litmus paper urine tests. Did you investigate to see whether the person's urine was more acid or alkaline?

REVICI: Yes, that was the first thing I did.* We know that urinary pH varies from person to person, but I could not find anything written in the entire literature of science about the correspondence of urinary pH to any other phenomena. It seemed that no one had ever asked the question: "What factor of the body or in the blood corresponds to the acid/base level of the urine?" So I began to study with laboratory dogs.

I used a catheter so that I could extract, for one to three minutes, just enough urine for electronic analysis of pH. Simultaneously, I also extracted blood. I was collecting blood and urine at the same time, under the same conditions, every half hour to an hour. First I measured the pH of both the urine and blood. Then, in analyzing the blood further, I measured the so-called alkaline-combining power, corresponding to the carbonates in the blood. I also meas-

---

* Today, Dr. Revici relies largely on variations of his patients' body temperature as a means of determining the acid or alkaline nature of a condition. He has discovered that a fever is an anabolic response to a catabolic condition, and thus treats such a condition with medications that have an anabolic effect. The opposite is also true. Revici has discovered that a lowered body temperature signals the body's catabolic response to an anabolic imbalance, and thus serves as a basis for therapeutic use of antianabolic agents.

ured the amount of chlorides and potassium in the blood every half hour. Because of such frequent extractions of both blood and urine, it was easy to make a series of curves illustrating all of the variations I found.

BRYANT: Were you looking for a correspondence between urinary pH and the pH of the blood?

REVICI: Exactly. But, in spite of extensive experimentation, I could find no correlation. Then I realized: in the blood, only a part of the base and alkaline substances are free. A sizeable percentage is bound with buffering proteins, which keep the blood from becoming too base or too alkaline. However, in the urine, the body has no more need to buffer anything; the urine has no function. It is simply eliminated, whether greatly base or greatly alkaline. This is part of the reason for such a discrepancy between the pH in urine and in blood.

With this in mind, I decided to measure the titrimetric alkalinity—including all of the alkaline substances which are free to react—of the blood. My measurements included both the ionized and buffered alkalinity of the blood, bound to proteins. All in all, I was able to measure total alkalinity in the blood, a measurement which had not been made before. And it was very clear that the variation in urinary pH corresponded perfectly with that of the total titrimetric alkalinity of the blood.

BRYANT: How did you use this information in working with your patients?

REVICI: First, I simply tried to correlate the variation of pain's intensity with variation in pH. In order to do this, I asked my patients for hourly urine samples, and to write down how their pain felt, not just at the moment of urinating, but during that entire, previous hour. Using scales of 0 - 10 designating a range of sensation from "no pain" to "unbearable pain," the patients recorded whether their pain had increased or decreased hour by hour and by how much. This information was correlated with the hourly analysis of their urine.

In this way, I obtained curves of the changing intensity of pain and of pH, indicating as well the changing titrimetric alkalinity of the blood. During this investigation I found a correspondence between increased alkalinity and increased pain among the patients who experienced pain during the evening. When the pH went down and their urine showed more acidity, their pain decreased. In contrast, among those who experienced morning pain, we saw a correspondence between acidity, a lowered pH, and increased pain.

BRYANT: So then you had an even better understanding of the correlation between eating and pain.

REVICI: Yes. Alkaline pain was increased after eating, when the body was experiencing the alkaline tide. Those who experienced the morning, acid pain, after fasting for seven to twelve hours, were relieved by the temporary alkalinity which they experienced directly after eating.

BRYANT: You actually showed two types of pain.

REVICI: Yes—one increasing when the body becomes acid; one increasing when the body becomes alkaline. This was the first time that a dualism related to acid/base balance was recognized as operating in the body.

BRYANT: Does pain respond to changes in the body, or do certain kinds of pain actually make the body more acid or more alkaline?

REVICI: I resolved that question by giving patients sodium bicarbonate, an alkaline substance. Immediately afterward, patients who experienced acid pain—morning pain—felt relief in the sites of their lesions, and their urine became less acid. Those who experienced alkaline or evening pain felt an increase in pain after taking the bicarbonate, and their urine too became even less acid. Next I administered phosphoric acid or mono-ammonium phosphate to both groups of patients. As could be expected, the acid pain increased, alkaline pain decreased, and urine showed a lower pH.

BRYANT: So you were able to see how those changes in the acid/base balance of the body actually produced or lessened pain in localized areas.

REVICI: Yes, and I came to the conclusion that the intensity of pain was a direct result of the acid/base balance in the body.

   Since pain itself was seen to be a response of a localized lesion to an acid or alkaline condition of the body, it appeared logical that the lesion itself might be either acid or alkaline, according to its nature and the variation of acid/base balance.

BRYANT: How were you able to measure the pH of lesions themselves?

REVICI: In the case of a patient with a large tumor of the face, characterized by acid pain, I made a small incision and inserted a little glass electrode to measure local pH. In normal tissue to which we had introduced the same electrode, pH had measured 7.35 - 7.37. However, I was amazed to see that here, at the site of acid pain, pH measured as low as 5.5. Nobody had ever reported finding such acidity anywhere in the body, except in the stomach. My results were so dramatically far from normal that I didn't even dare to publish my findings until many confirmations had been repeated.

BRYANT: What other cases did you document?

REVICI: The next patient I worked with had alkaline pain caused by a breast carcinoma. I repeated the same procedure, and the results were just as dramatic. The lesion of this patient measured 8, showing an abnormal level of alkalinity. When I administered sodium bicarbonate, the local pH level rose to a shocking 8.8, and the alkaline pain increased.

I concluded from this that pathological pain is produced directly by a local acidosis or a local alkalosis.

BRYANT: But what actually causes one lesion to be of an acid character, and another to be alkaline to begin with?

REVICI: In starting to study, I consulted the existing medical literature and found that Otto Warburg of Germany had shown that anoxybiotic metabolism—without oxygen—produces lactic acid. Immediately I set out to see if my patients with acid pain had, locally or generally, more lactic acid than the others.

First I found a boy with an enormous tumor of the knee. I took blood from the efferent veins and found that in general, his blood was high in lactic acid. Then I took blood when he was in very severe pain, and I found higher amounts of lactic acid. This corroborated the work of Otto Warburg.

BRYANT: What about alkaline pain?

REVICI: I searched the literature as thoroughly as I could, but I could not find one single work in existence which addressed the problem of alkalosis. So I continued studying. From a patient with alkaline pain from a breast tumor, I took fluid running from a lesion and I found sodium carbonate and sodium bicarbonate in it.

BRYANT: Where were these substances being generated?

REVICI: I concluded that they were coming from the salt in her body—because in this case, the chloride was fixed, and the sodium was remaining free to bond with carbonic ions, yielding the alkaline substance. The next step was to find and to show that locally, in the site of alkaline pain, there is a retention of chlorides.

BRYANT: How did you show that?

REVICI: I did an autopsy of a cancer patient of mine who had just died. I took this patient's tumor and measured the amount of chlorides in the tumor itself. I then compared this amount with the amount in other, normal tissues of the body. This patient had experienced alkaline pain, and the lesion demonstrated a local alkalosis. In fact, this lesion contained between six and eight times more chlorine than in the normal tissue.

So it appeared clear, and I later demonstrated through further measurements of lesion biopsies, that the alkaline pain comes from locally fixed chlorine, while sodium remains free to bond carbonic anions. This contributes greatly to the formation of alkaline substances and conditions.

Clearly then, I had determined that pathological pain is a dualistic phenomenon. We can no longer talk about the existence of just one kind of pathological pain.

BRYANT: What about treatment? Did you begin to administer acid and alkaline substances in order to acidify or alkalinize the body chemistry?

REVICI: Yes. We administered a medication called Coramine first, and noticed that, as a result, alkaline pain decreased while acid pain increased. Then I administered other substances, including soy sauce. We observed that acid pain decreased as a result, while alkaline pain increased. Since it was clear that the two kinds of pain responded as opposites to the same medication, my discoveries left the realm of theory; they would soon be applied.

We had finally been led to a means of combating pain without relying on morphine derivatives or other narcotics which work upon the nervous system. This experimentation, in fact, led to the discovery of an entire series of substances which would work to eliminate either acid pain or alkaline pain.

Of course, the acid/alkaline reaction is really not just telling us how to treat the pain itself. It is telling us how to treat the condition which causes the pain.

BRYANT: I sense a joy about the work you've done as a research scientist and as a physician to ease pain in the world.

REVICI: Yes, ever since I was a child I have had the desire to help people. I learned from my father, especially — a physician who was deeply loved and respected by everyone. He never said no to a patient in distress. He would leave the house at three or four in the morning to see someone who needed him.

I was encouraged very early on, as a child, to learn and to experiment. And in fact, in my youth I had performed many experiments to show the antagonism between fatty acids and sterols.

BRYANT: Which brings us back to acid and alkaline pain. What were the substances which you discovered to eliminate pain?

REVICI: First I wanted to see if acid and alkaline types of pain correlated with two classes of lipids: sterols and fatty acids.

Fortunately, I had the opportunity to study tissue, during autopsies, from patients at our hospitals in Mexico and in New York. I had attended these patients, and I knew whether their pain had been alkaline or acid. In studying, I found that in patients with alkaline pain, chlorides were bound to fatty acids in the lesions, leaving sodium free to bond with carbonic anions and giving us the alkaline carbonates and bicarbonates. The patients who had suffered from acid pain showed a high amount of sterols in the lesions. This led me to study the lipids further, and I correlated my understanding of pain's own dualism with the basic antagonism between these two types of lipidic substances: fatty acids and sterols.

BRYANT: What was your next step?

REVICI: I realized early on that a satisfying definition of lipids did not exist in the medical literature. Certainly the definition "a fatty acid or fatty-acid derivative" was not sufficient, and definitions which described the effects of "greasiness," for instance, were broad enough to include non-lipidic substances such as paraffin. Nor was I satisfied with the definition of lipid as "a substance which is more soluble in neutral solvent than in water."

BRYANT: How did you go about investigating the essential qualities of lipids?

REVICI: First, I utilized the results of some studies of the forces present in various substances. I knew of the polar groups — groups of atoms characterized by positively or negatively charged, electrostatic forces — and I compared polar substances — such as water, hydrochloric acid, and alkaline substances made up of two or more polar groups bound together — with nonpolar substances such as the hydrocarbons. These remain without polar groups.

Surprisingly, however, when I investigated the properties of lipids, I found that they comprise both polar and nonpolar substances — having a polar group bound to a nonpolar group. This was an important characteristic, in the sense that a polar group will make a substance soluble in water, while the nonpolar group makes a substance insoluble in water.

I was then able to identify *lipids* as polar/nonpolar substances in which the nonpolar forces are greater than the electrostatic forces of the polar groups.

BRYANT: So you actually redefined the lipids!

REVICI: Yes, and with this definition we have a new level of lipidic systematization. You see, a polar group can be either positive or negative. So, depending on the predominance, we have positive and negative lipids. Positive lipids, the sterols, are associated with anabolic activity. Negative lipids, the fatty acids, are associated with catabolic activity.

Fatty acids form easily penetrable membranes, while the sterols resist penetration. As a result, a predominance of sterols causes cells to lack oxygen. This causes the formation of anoxybiotic lactic acid in the body, and thus, acid pain. Conversely, in the case of alkaline pain, we have a predominance of fatty acids, in which membrane penetration and metabolism are free; plus, we have a lot of oxygen, inducing oxidation.

BRYANT: So, within the dualistic model of pain that you'd discovered, you found that different lipidic agents could reduce both alkaline and acid pain?

REVICI: Yes. And lipids are ideal agents because of their stability, due primarily to their insolubility in water. This insolubility forms a group apart from all water-soluble constituents. Lipids are able to function without continuous interference from other constituents. Hydrosolubility and rapidity of reactions among most electrolytes, proteins and even carbohydrates made these other substances far less desirable.

I set up many experiments for doctors, showing the results of administering fatty acids and sterols to patients in pain. When sterols were given to a person with acid pain, we all witnessed an increase in the patient's pain. When sterols were given to a person in alkaline pain, the pain decreased sharply. The opposite effects were experienced through the administration of fatty acids. These experiments showed how two categories of lipids have opposite effects in cases of alkaline and acid pain.

BRYANT: It seems that your desire to understand pathological pain led to a number of discoveries. Could you sum up your work in this field, briefly?

REVICI: In review, I showed the existence, clinically, of morning and evening pain. Acid pain responded well to food, while alkaline pain actually caused a fear of food. I also showed the correspondence between urinary pH and titrimetric alkalinity of the blood. I identified local acidosis and local alkalosis as sources of acid and alkaline types of pain. And I showed the correlation between these two classes of pain and the substances (sodium carbonate or sodium bicarbonate) which aggravate alkaline pain and alleviate acid pain; the reverse was true for lactic acid, which aggravates acid pain and alleviates alkaline pain. This proved that acid and alkaline pain respond in opposite ways to the same substance.

Finally I worked to define the lipids. This work led me to show how reducing the permeability of a lipidic membrane — characteristic of sterols — slows down oxidation, and how increasing such permeability speeds up oxidation. I also justified the use of lipids on a clinical basis.

We have shown that certain metabolisms produce acids such as lactic acid, and other metabolisms produce alkaline substances.

BRYANT: Then it seems that if you could work directly with the metabolism itself, you would be much closer to working on the cause of the problem rather than just the symptoms.

REVICI: Certainly, it is more efficient and much more beautiful to work on the factor which *produces* the local acidosis or alkalosis — its cause — than it is to work directly on the local condition itself.

BRYANT: Are the lipids actually capable of correcting the conditions which cause imbalance?

REVICI: Yes. That is my interest. We have found that lipids, in the form of sterols and fatty acids, are extremely effective agents in treating a great variety of problems, including pain. Today, more than fifty years after I began working to understand these problems, I still administer anti-fatty acid or anti-sterol preparations, which affect the acid/alkaline balance of the entire body, and not just the lesion or problem area. Also, I am still administering sodium carbonate and sodium bicarbonate, phosphoric acid, or monoammonium phospate with great success when testing to determine the kind of pain present.

BRYANT: Can you talk about how your work in the field of pain can be applied to other health conditions as well?

REVICI: At the Institute we have applied the principle of anabolic/acid or catabolic/alkaline conditions to other forms of distress. Itching, for instance, shows a correspondence with either an alkaline or acid condition. There is a recognizable difference be-

tween itching which is caused by an acid condition and that which
is caused by an alkaline one.

Very interesting also is my work with vertigo. I have shown the
difference between a vertigo caused by acidity and alkalinity. In
fact, this work has been mentioned in the AMA's publication, *Applied Otolaryngology.*

Another application of these same principles can be seen in the
diagnosis and treatment of two types of hearing impairment. One
is acid; the other is alkaline. Each type of impairment is exaggerated by a state of acidity or alkalinity in the body.

BRYANT: Has your work been applied at all in the treatment of
psychological imbalance or mental illness?

REVICI: Yes. The acid/base relationship to psychological disease
is very interesting. I recall one case of a young boy who was manic
in his behavior. His father, who was devoted to him, was greatly
disturbed by his son's vacillations between states of fury and states
of absolute calm. So I suggested that we make the same experiment which I had made in learning about pain. I asked to have
a sample of the boy's urine every hour during a period of ten hours.
And I asked his father to observe the behavior of the boy during
every hour, and to rate his behavior on a scale of one to ten so
that I could determine whether the problem was due to an acid
condition or an alkaline one.

After twenty-four hours, his father returned to me with about
fourteen urine samples and a list of his changing behavior throughout the day, rated on a scale of one to ten. A rating of ten showed
that the boy was really crazy, and a one showed him being extremely
calm. So we were able to make an entire curve of his behavior along
with a curve showing the pH of his urine.

It was really impressive. Whenever the boy's pH became more
acid, he became more agitated. The opposite was also true. When
his urine showed alkalinity, the boy showed perfect calm. It was
one of the most beautifully clear correspondences I had ever seen.

BRYANT: Did you treat him with alkaline substances?

REVICI: I administered both acid and alkaline substances. As
you've suspected, giving him sodium bicarbonate made him perfectly calm for hours. On the contrary, when I gave him phosphoric
acid or mono-ammonium phosphate, he became quite agitated,
confirming, in this case, that a condition that had been considered psychological was actually biological in origin.

This completed one phase of my study of acid and alkaline abnormalities and symptoms, starting with the pain and going to the phenomenon of itching, and then to vertigo, impaired hearing, and finally to a physical disorder which manifested as what could be considered a psychological problem.

BRYANT: As a biochemist, you actually compound your own medicinal substances. Do most of these substances reflect the principles you've been discussing today?

REVICI: Yes. At the Institute we use anabolic and catabolic agents, chemically well-defined agents of many different natures which have an anabolic/acid effect, or a catabolic/basic effect.

The medicines are administered in capsules or in drops, most often. Occasionally, injections are necessary.

BRYANT: Your story has given me new insights into the science of balance, which seems to be the science most desperately needed for the future of our entire planet.

REVICI: It's good to remember that we are in symbiosis with millions and millions of entities. My own interest in astronomy, the contemplation of billions of suns, has shown me how small we are. We are independent, but most importantly, we are interrelated beings. Just think. We have billions of cells, every day dying, every day being created. Each cell contains countless inactive genes, active genes, a nucleus, endoplasm and a membrane. It is born, it lives, it functions, it dies. Individual cells, we might think, are living independent, individual lives. But we should allow ourselves to truly understand that each one of us individual, "independent" beings is formed by the symbiosis of millions of cells. Mutual dependence—that is the pattern. Nothing more, nothing less.

AN EAST-WEST DIALOGUE

DRS. TROGAWA RINPOCHE & EMANUEL REVICI, M.D.

Although he has worked in the context of Western research laboratories and has never studied Oriental philosophy or medicine, Dr. Revici's observation of anabolic and catabolic processes in metabolism has been compared to the Eastern principle of Yin (roughly, expanding), and Yang (contracting). His in-depth, often abstruse work in the field of biochemistry gives scientific weight to ancient ways of approaching science and medicine, just as thousands of years of Oriental medical tradition serve to validate some of his scientific work.

Dr. Trogawa is a practitioner of traditional Tibetan medicine. Born in Lhasa, Tibet in 1929, he was raised in a monastery where he studied Buddhism and meditation. He began medical studies at the age of sixteen as an apprentice to a renowned physician in Lhasa. This apprenticeship lasted nine years. His studies involved memorizing the classic medical texts as well as learning physical therapies and traditional diagnostic techniques such as urinalysis and sphygmology— pulse analysis—plus pharmacopoeia and pharmaceutical manufacture, including the most esoteric aspect of Tibetan medicine: the making of the Jewel Medicines.

In 1956 Dr. Trogawa moved to Sikkim, where he practiced medicine. In 1963 he became the teaching master at the Tibetan Medical Institute in Dharamsala, India. In 1983, he came to the West for the first time in order to participate in the first conference on Tibetan Medicine in Venice, Italy. Since then, he has lectured extensively in North American Buddhist teaching centers on the philosophy and history of Tibetan medicine. His talks include information on Tibetan approaches to diagnosis and healing using urinalysis, diet, herbs, minerals, spiritual practice, and many other aspects of the ancient

165

medical system.

Dr. Trogawa has shown a great deal of interest in learning about Western science, philosophy and technology. And although Dr. Revici's training has been completely conventional as a Western scientist, his interest in quantum physics and years of independent experimentation have brought him toward a recognition of balance as a principle of health. This is the fundamental basis for their mutual understanding.

The following dialogue (Shakia Dorje, interpretor) is an expression of Dr. Trogawa's sincere desire to communicate with Western scientists and medical practitioners.

INTRODUCTION

On Thanksgiving Day, 1984, my twin brother Bruce called from Los Angeles to tell me about Dr. Trogawa, who is renowned not only as a Tibetan medical doctor, but also as a meditation master. He had recently given a lecture in Los Angeles, and would soon be teaching in New York, so I made plans to attend several lectures. That same winter, I was interviewing Dr. Emanuel Revici. I described to Dr. Trogawa, as best I could, the priorities and development of Dr. Revici's work over a sixty-five-year period. When I suggested that Dr. Revici's method might serve as a bridge between Oriental and Occidental approaches to medicine, Dr. Trogawa expressed great interest in exchanging ideas with him. He seemed to be especially impressed with Dr. Revici's advanced age (eighty-eight at the time of our meeting) and his dedication to helping people.

Dr. Revici eagerly awaited the meeting. He asked numerous questions about the "lama doctor," and did his best to translate my brief impressions of the Tibetan medical system into data he could interpret scientifically. In answer to his questions, I explained that Tibetan medicine was greatly dependent upon herbs and other natural substances, and that surgery was not used except in extreme cases. We spoke about the psychological aspects of mantra, meditation and prayer. He compared this concept with work done by Dr. Lawrence LeShan, one of the first Western scientists to investigate the relationship between personality and illness during the 1950s and '60s. After several conversations, Dr. Revici exclaimed, "Tibet is an oasis! The Tibetans have been living with an ancient culture isolated from the rest of the world by the Himalayan Range. We have much to learn from them!" Dr. Revici's interest and professional curiosity, as well as his ability to think critically about a system as unique as Tibetan medicine, gave me great confidence in the importance and relevance of the upcoming cross-cultural dialogue.

The two doctors met for the first time at Dr. Revici's office and later at his home. An elegant European gentleman, Dr. Revici showed fascination and respect for the doctor in burgundy-colored monk's robes. Dr. Trogawa's presence reflected great mindfulness and attention. The interview itself was an expression of mutual interest and respect.

DIALOGUE

BRYANT: Today's discussion offers us an opportunity to witness the meeting of two very different medical systems. You each work within your own medical tradition. However, Dr. Trogawa, you've been separated from your homeland since 1956 and now work in exile, mostly in India. And you, Dr. Revici, have chosen to develop a scientific course which takes your medical practice beyond allopathic medicine.

REVICI: It is an honor to be here with you, discussing the differences and similarities between two systems of science and medicine.

In my research over the years, I've found that all pathology and disease is a product of either catabolic (destructive, breaking down) or anabolic (constructive, building up) activity, unchecked. Even pain can be characterized as either catabolic or anabolic. At the Institute of Applied Biology, we have learned to utilize anabolic or "building up" agents against catabolic pain and disease. We use catabolic or "breaking down" agents against anabolic pain and disease.

TROGAWA: In the Tibetan medical system, we recognize two types of energy or activity: strengthening or growing activity, and declining or destructive activity. In Chinese and Japanese medicine, these two types of energy are generally categorized as Yin and Yang. It would seem that we are working with very similar principles. Also, it seems that we use a similar approach in determining which medicines to use. We use strengthening, building medicines against the declining or destructive conditions, and we use destructive or declining medicines against conditions of overabundance. Our system is over a thousand years old.

REVICI: Perhaps we have even more in common. For instance, here at the Institute we have learned to always approach each medical problem in its entirety, rather than to simply match up a specific substance with a particular set of symptoms. We have found that every case of a disease has a different character. One case of breast cancer may be anabolic in nature; another may be catabolic. Vertigo, eczema... every health problem is an individual health problem. Each one may be anabolic or catabolic, and the nature of a problem may change during treatment. Therapy must be applied accordingly.

Of course, the basic concept we're working with is dualism—two opposite manifestations of two opposite forces. All manifestations in nature, including disease, are simply part of this movement between destructive and constructive characters, catabolic and anabolic. At the Institute of Applied Biology, our entire system of analysis and treatment is based on what I have just described.

In treating disease, first we determine which force characterizes the disease at the time of diagnosis. Then we administer the most appropriate anabolic medication for a particular case of catabolic disease, or vice versa. In the case of cancer, our first objective has always been to stop the pain first; next, slowly reduce the tumor.

However, during a treatment, due either to the condition's progress or to the treatment itself, the disease may change to its opposite in character. When this happens, medication must change accordingly. For this reason, we must constantly monitor the status of a disease. We call our approach "guided therapy," therapy guided by analysis. We practice this therapy, in part, by making frequent analyses of the urine. This method may be applied to any condition.

TROGAWA: This is similar to a principle of our practice, wherein we are continually re-examining the patient and continually adjusting our medication.

REVICI: At the Institute, we have been successful in treating cancer with this method over the past fifty years. During that time, the substances we've used and our methods of diagnosis have become more and more efficacious. And since I am a physical chemist as well as a physician, part of my work is to synthesize almost all of the substances I use.

I've described the basis of our approach, but there are many other factors. For instance, we're interested in observing the level of biological organization that is being attacked by a disease. A disease will attack only one level of biological organization at a time. It may attack at the genetic level, at the level of the cell, at the level of the tissue or at the organ level. And each medical agent only works at one specific level of organization.

For Western people used to identifying a group of related symptoms as one particular disease, and used to treating that group of symptoms with one specific medication, it is difficult to accept my view that every disease is an individual case, to be analyzed individually. It is hard for people to understand, for instance, that there is not just one substance which treats cancer successfully.

TROGAWA: Your way of approaching disease is very much in accordance with the Buddha Dharma teachings, starting with the basic duality in which we find ourselves: subject and object, the overabundant and destructive nature of our world—our reality.

REVICI: How would you describe the main approach of Tibetan medicine?

TROGAWA: For mild disorders, we give dietary as well as certain behavioral instructions. This can suffice if a disease is not too serious. If the disease is more serious, we will begin to treat it with herbs or minerals, or a number of natural medicines. These medicines can be prepared in a great variety of ways. In some cases, the doses are very small, more or less corresponding to the miniscule doses of homeopathy. In cases of serious disorders, the dosages are much stronger. In finishing a treatment, we might cauterize.

We treat different types of cancer differently. In breast cancer, I use herbal compounds which are cooked as decoctions and drunk by the patients. I also use a mantra[1] in conjunction with this. In a mild case of cancer of the root of the tongue, I have had success using medicine exclusively, without a mantra.

REVICI: In general, the majority of your medicines come from plants? From minerals? From chemicals?

TROGAWA: The majority are from plants. Some are from minerals, precious stones and metals. We use gold, silver, and mercury, for instance. It all depends upon the condition of the patient.

Sometimes we use animal products as well, such as rhinoceros horn, bezoar[2], musk, bear's bile—also deer antler, other kinds of horn, and certain kinds of flesh and blood, most of which must come from wild animals.

REVICI: Do you say, "This plant or this animal substance is always good for this disease"? Or does each case demand a special, unique treatment?

TROGAWA: We can sometimes treat many different cases of a disease as one entity, using one substance as medicine, but there are many other ways to think about the medicinal properties of plants and their relationship to illness. For instance, the same plant, prepared in different ways, has different properties; different parts of one plant may have very different properties; and plants, once combined with other plants or substances, also have different properties. So the way in which plants and other substances are

---

[1]*Mantra:* a sound meditation, usually the repetition of a syllable or syllables which represents and brings about a certain state of mind.

[2]*Bezoar:* a concretion found in the digestive system of elephants, cows and other ruminants.

combined is very important. The medications we use are of varying strengths depending upon the disease in question.

REVICI: Can most of the plants you use be found in North America or Europe?

TROGAWA: A number of our medicinal plants seem to be exclusively native to Tibet. Some grow only in very high altitudes, near the snow line. We are finding many more plants in India now. Many of these are rare plants which must be picked in certain types of environments during a specific time of year.

REVICI: It would be very interesting to study some of the plants native to Tibet—those which you find to be especially medicinal.

TROGAWA: From a modern scientific point of view, I certainly agree. His Holiness the Dalai Lama has initiated a project to produce a very special product, which we call the Jewel Medicine. This is now being made in large quantities in the hope of its benefiting people all over the world. These medicines are based on one particular substance used in combination with many other medications.

REVICI: I would very much like to learn about your system of diagnosis and treatment. Can you make an introduction to this topic?

TROGAWA: In the question of diagnosis, we are first concerned with the details of information which are found through the pulse. We examine the crucial points, which correspond to the organs of the body. Urine analysis comes next. We also observe the tongue and the eyes, and we listen carefully to the verbal information given by the patient to find out what effects certain foods might have had on him or her while ill, or what kinds of thoughts or feelings have presented themselves anew during the period of illness.

REVICI: What about changes in symptoms throughout the day, at different times? Have you discovered that a patient may feel better in the morning or in the evening?

TROGAWA: Yes, the time when one vomits or has pain is very important in our diagnostic system. But in order to go more deeply into this discussion, one must understand that we base our diagnosis on the status of the three humors[3] in the body.

---

[3]*Humors*: principles of energy categorized as "wind," "bile," and "phlegm." Each is associated with specific organs as well as physical and psychological conditions. For more detailed information, see Appendix *Tibetan Medicine*, especially the section on "Elements & Humors."

The first of these is the *wind* humor, associated with the element air. Should one be suffering from a disease of wind, one's pain will be augmented at three or four in the morning, before daybreak, and before dusk in the afternoon.

Should a patient be suffering from a fire or *bile* disorder, perhaps with hypertension, the patient will feel an augmentation of symptoms at the middle of the day and at midnight.

The humor *phlegm* is basically associated with the elements earth and water. A person with a phlegmatic disorder will have a worsening of symptoms in the morning or after sunset.

Then there are other considerations in the fluctuation of a disease. For instance, if the disease is moving in the direction of enfeeblement, it will present itself more strongly in the morning. If the disease is in the direction of excess, it will present itself more strongly in the evening. Then there are even more fluctuations we consider in a day, but those are the two basic ones we consider.

REVICI: What you say concurs strongly with my own findings. Catabolic pain is stronger in the morning. Anabolic pain is stronger in the evening. Now, what role does food play in treatment?

TROGAWA: Food is very important in our treatment. Once a patient is ill, we must consider diet, and the more ill the patient is, the more stringent the diet will become. We give dietary instruction to most of our patients.

A food's relative heating or cooling property is the primary consideration. Heating foods are appropriate for people with a cooling disorder; cooling foods are appropriate for someone with an overheating disorder.

On a relative scale, all foods are either more heating or more cooling. Some are very close to an equilibrium.

REVICI: Am I correct in assuming that the diseases themselves are also considered either cooling or heating according to the symptoms?

TROGAWA: Yes. When I diagnose a patient, the first question I ask is whether the patient is suffering from a heating or a cooling disorder. Then another question I will address fairly quickly in the diagnosis is how intense or strong is the level of heat or cold. This will determine whether I treat the patient simply with diet, or with diet and behavioral instruction, or diet, behavioral instruction and medication, or with all these methods plus a spiritual application.

But this also depends upon where the disorder is concentrated in the body, and the disorder's stage of maturity.

REVICI: It would be helpful to give an example. Can you talk specifically about tuberculosis, for instance?

TROGAWA: Tuberculosis may be either a hot or cold disorder. We must first determine which kind of tuberculosis we are dealing with. Then we must find out whether it is attacking the lungs, the bones or the intestines. Is there a production of serous fluid in conjunction with the tuberculosis or not? According to all this information, we will begin to prescribe a medication.

REVICI: What is your rate of success in working with cancer?

TROGAWA: I have cured some conditions diagnosed as cancer by Western doctors' biopsies, but not a great number. However, I have effected many reprieves, which I consider successes, as well. There are many cases where a doctor has predicted only one month or two months of life left for the patient, and I have helped the patient to live many months or a year or longer, in reasonable health. Although they eventually die, their lives are extended using the traditional Tibetan methods.

It all depends, of course, on the severity of the disease. We have fairly good results with what is diagnosed in Western hospitals as being breast cancer. Tumors in general do not present too much of a problem for us. We have documented our capacity to cure these. But there is a much better chance of treating a patient successfully with Tibetan medicine if the patient has not received allopathic chemotherapy or radiation.

In Italy last year, it was reported to me that a patient I treated for a "hopeless" case of brain cancer had recovered satisfactorily. Furthermore, the patient had been treated unsuccessfully with surgery and chemotherapy and many other heavy treatments earlier. When I first saw her, she'd been given less than a month to live. Her treatment was strongly connected with the practice of Buddhism. It was attitude as much as medicine which made the significant difference. In many such cases, we resist medical treatment alone, and accompany the administration of medicine with mantra repetition and other spiritual practices.

REVICI: I am not very familiar with the Buddhist system. Could you describe the spiritual practices of your religion as they relate to medicine?

TROGAWA: In considering Buddhist practice and Tibetan medicine, we start with the basic duality of our subjective being and the objective world. It happens that our world is made of our per-

ceptual experience: vision, sound, touch, smell, taste. Subjective-
ly, we do not understand these conditions, but our minds seek explanations, so we have illusions about them. These are actually
delusions—reflections of the mind—but we tend to grasp at them
as if they were something which they are not. We tend to have
an artificial concept of them. Unknowingly, we create our own diseases through the continuous projection of false notions about our
experience.

Certainly then, in learning about the body, we must explore the
connection between body and mind. In accordance with our philosophy, we try to consider how the body manifests itself, and then,
in that circumstance, how the disease occurs. And we try to relate
to that condition through physical applications of medicine and
other levels of treatment. I also think it's important for the physician to have a proper outlook upon himself or herself as physician.

REVICI: In our research at the Institute, we have also pursued
an understanding of the relationship between the psychological
and the physical as applied to cancer and other disease. Dr. Lawrence LeShan, studied this topic for twelve years in our laboratory, in a scientific manner. He found that psychological conditions
have an enormous influence not only on the production of a disease but also on the disease's evolution, and even on its response
to a particular treatment.

I would be interested to know how much of your approach is
psychological or even religious as opposed to solely physical. Can
you describe, for instance, how you would treat breast cancer?

TROGAWA: Generally, for breast cancer I use medicine in conjunction with a mantra or incantation in order to bring about a
healing state of mind. For instance, Om Mani Padme Hum is a
mantra for compassion. Other mantras may represent qualities like
wisdom or purification. A mantra is a means of relaying psychological power through certain sounds.

We learn these sounds from the teachings of the Buddha or from
certain prophecies. They are all established in tradition. The physician meditates on Sange Menla, the Medicine Buddha, and learns
to utilize the power of the mantra through that meditation.

We use the sounds along with certain medicines to cure the disease. Then, as for results, there are two basic possibilities. If the
tumor is fairly small, it will shrink and disappear by itself. If the
tumor is somewhat larger, it will mature; then there will be an excretion of pus and so forth, and it will collapse.

REVICI: I see the thing psychologically. To me, your treatment

is related to the power of suggestion, which may have a good deal
to do with the patient's recovery. Certainly pain may be provoked
or alleviated through the power of suggestion. One can say to a
patient, "Your pain will be gone in a few days," and the pain may
go away through the power of suggestion alone. On the contrary,
we can say, "When you stand up, you will feel much pain." This
too will have an effect on the patient's physical state.

It is known that the power of suggestion can actually affect the
leukocytes in the body, altering the body's defense system as well
as other bodily functions. So I'm interested to see how much the
Tibetan physician, consciously and unconsciously, practices the
power of suggestion. Perhaps completely unconsciously, the doctor is establishing a connection between the psyche of the patient
and his own psyche.

TROGAWA: Yes, the mind is very powerful, in general. So if the
patient has a sense of confidence in the physician, and if the physician has a truly positive and loving attitude toward a patient, that
alone has a certain value in the curative process, and certainly mag-
nifies the effect of one's treatment.

Some people with cancer have practiced Buddhist meditation
and, without using any medication, have actually cured themselves.
We believe that everything is interconnected — that everything is
supported by everything else. So our Buddhist philosophy certainly
has a large role to play in medicine.

REVICI: I am not involved with religion, but I am interested to
find out how you would describe *post mortem* existence from the
Buddhist point of view.

TROGAWA: We are born into the continuous process of existence, and as we are born, we go through the inevitable process
of growing up and growing old, which leads eventually to dying.
It is a cyclic process. We believe that after death a person is born
in another lifetime, and after that, another lifetime, and again and
again.

Immediately after dying, the person enters the intermediate
stage, the *bardo* stage, between one lifetime and the next. There
is no physical existence in the bardo state. But there is mind: consciousness and feeling. And so there is pleasure and pain.

Most people are drawn into a new life with new parents by the
force of their own *karma,* which they have created themselves according to the acts of their past lives.

REVICI: Your brief description of the Tibetan medical system has certainly given me a great deal to think about, especially in terms of the bonds between psychology and physiology.

TROGAWA: This is for you—a picture of the Buddha of Medicine. He is the primordial founder of Tibetan medicine, who existed long before our world began, and who taught the primordial teachings of medicine. The Medicine Buddha is blue-colored like the sky because his knowledge is all-pervading. Also, the Medicine Buddha has the power of aspiration. So if a person is favorably inclined toward the Medicine Buddha, there is an intuitive contact, which gives a power to that individual as well.

   I will pronounce the sound which is the name of the Medicine Buddha. The sounds alone may benefit many people with many different conditions of disease. It is a general medicine mantra: TA YA TA / OM BE KAN DZE / BE KAN DZE / MA HA BE KAN DZE / RA DZA / SA MUNG GA TE / SO HA

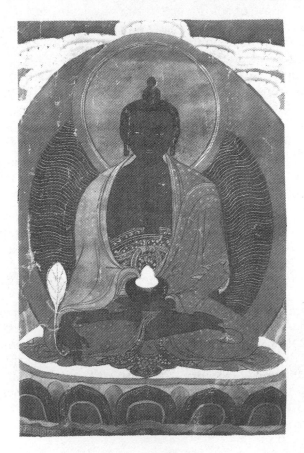

A Scientist's View of Human Potential

JACOB ZIGHELBOIM, M.D.

Jacob Zighelboim, M.D. is an Associate Professor of Medicine and Immunology at the UCLA School of Medicine. In the late 1960s he worked in Israel and Venezuela, investigating autoimmune disease and immune reactions to transplanted organs. In 1972 he began to pursue a fellowship in immunology at UCLA, and was drawn to study immunological approaches to cancer treatment. As a scientist and physician, he began to explore the roles of vaccines derived from tumor cells and tumor-cell extracts, as well as bacterial agents and biologic-response modifiers — drugs which reinforce the immune system.

In 1983, Dr. Zighelboim discovered he had lymphoma. After treatment with radiation therapy, he took a sabbatical from UCLA and began looking into psychological factors as they are related to the cause and resolution of cancer and other disorders. Today he is fully committed to the development of integrated approaches to healing. He offers week-long conferences called Healing the Self, which give participants a chance to discover and call upon various personal resources in relation to their own healing processes. Techniques and activities are drawn from his scientific background and medical training in the fields of hematology, oncology, immunology, microbiology and psychology, as well as techniques of exploring consciousness, such as meditation and dream counseling. Dr. Zighelboim has published over eighty articles in scientific journals and contributed to many medical and scientific books.

INTRODUCTION

During the first six years of my investigation of cancer, I con-
tacted several doctors working in the field of chemotherapy, ranging from the National Cancer Institute's chief of surgery to the
clinical director of NYU Medical Center, as well as physicians from
several institutions, including Memorial Sloan-Kettering Cancer
Center, Maimonides, Mt. Sinai and Columbia Presbyterian Hospitals in New York City. All declined to enter the dialogue.

In 1986 I discussed this curious situation with a physician friend
who suggested that I get in touch with Dr. Jacob Zighelboim at
the UCLA Medical Center. "Not only is he an oncologist working
in the field of immunology," my friend told me, "he's also a cancer
patient." When Dr. Zighelboim and I met, I began to describe in
some detail the various points of view explored throughout the
book. But before I could finish, Dr. Zighelboim asked, "Just what
view are you trying to promote?"

I explained then that my purpose was not to proffer any particular point of view, but rather to present various perspectives in
the form of a cross-cultural forum. "With a full understanding of
our individual needs and values," I said, "and a broad view of the
resources available to us, we can each develop a method of treatment including several levels of therapy, ranging from chemotherapy or radiation to diet, meditation and herbs." "Well," he countered.
"The book itself will come to represent a specific point of view,
and someone or some group of people is bound not to like it. You
can't help but alienate someone." Then smiling, he added, "But
that's okay. Turn the tape recorder on."

I was impressed with Dr. Zighelboim's personal journey through
the medical establishment, his "take charge" attitude, his own personal confrontation with cancer, and most of all, his personal growth
as a patient living with cancer, open to discovering the subtle interplay among mind, disease and medicine. He has met a tremendous challenge, and he has used this challenge as a catalyst for
exploring personal healing—his own and that of others.

DIALOGUE

BRYANT: Can you describe cancer and cancer treatment from an immunologist's perspective?

ZIGHELBOIM: From my perspective, the cancer process represents a disturbance — an alteration at the genetic level. This alteration may be closely related to changes in the genetic material, or perhaps it's more closely related to the development of new growth patterns in response to altered surroundings. It's not just that one particular gene becomes active when it shouldn't. It's an interplay of multiple factors — a very complex transformational process which causes the cell to behave in a particular way — which we call cancer.

BRYANT: What are the effects of this transformation? How do cancer cells act differently from other cells?

ZIGHELBOIM: The characteristic of cancer cells which makes the cancer process so serious is the cancer cells' tendency to remain immature. Cancer cells replicate but do not undergo their full differentiation. Their development is arrested. The dangerous thing is that since they don't mature, they don't die off. This leads to an accumulation of cells. Death is part of cells' normal development and life cycle. The cell should reach a point of senescence, and then die. If cancer cells died when their time came, there would be no cancer as we know it.

BRYANT: So the immunologist approaches cancer not so much as an invader, but as the effect of an aberrant process of some sort.

ZIGHELBOIM: Yes. The ideal way to effect resolution of the problem is to repair the defect. We want to stimulate the cell to mature in a normal pattern and undergo its natural path of development. That's why molecular biology and biologic approaches to cancer therapy involve using hormones or biologically active molecules, which have the capacity to facilitate the development of the cell.

Several biologic methods are aimed toward helping the cells to mature, in order that they may die off as part of a natural cycle. As long as cancer cells have a capacity to die as a natural part of their life cycle, they don't represent a problem or a threat to the survival of the individual. But if the stem cells — the cancer cells which have the capacity to keep dividing and reproducing — self-perpetuate, the cancer is fed indefinitely.

BRYANT: Does science know anything about the effects of diet on these stem cells?

ZIGHELBOIM: No, because first of all, we don't know how to isolate stem cells. We know they're there, and we have several technologies to prove their presence, but we don't have enough markers to identify them correctly and to separate them. We do know that diets high in fat will promote certain cancers. In animals, we can affect the incidence of cancer and the rate of tumor growth through diet.

We also know that in humans, certain cancers correlate with dietary habits. But even without direct evidence of diet's effect on stem cells, I think most people agree that, in general, diet is an important variable that has to be given more attention, especially as a measure toward preventing certain cancers.

BRYANT: How does the immunological approach to cancer treatment relate to the more commonly used cytotoxic-chemotherapy approach?

ZIGHELBOIM: Cytotoxic chemotherapy is a very different approach. It's based upon the premise that there is a foreign entity in the body which needs to be destroyed by very aggressive, radical approaches. In many circumstances, the chemotherapy approach is not harmonious or congruent with immunological processes. In fact, we know that chemotherapy can damage the immune system. It's an approach directed specifically to the cancer cell. It's based on the idea that the cancer cell must be destroyed or killed, and that we need to use a powerful drug to do it.

BRYANT: Why do you think we've chosen to react to cancer by using a method which can actually damage the immune system?

ZIGHELBOIM: Historically, there are few examples of cooperative approaches to dealing with what we perceive to be foreign threats to our existence. Such threats are almost always handled in militaristic ways. So it's not surprising that the same approach is used in medicine. Since the beginning, cancer has been likened to diseases caused by foreign invaders such as bacteria and germs. Germs are treated with chemicals called antibiotics; since cancer is not susceptible to antibiotics, we've developed different substances along the same lines. They're aggressive drugs, consonant with the way we handle what we perceive to be foreign threats. We want to kill the cancer—to destroy the enemy and take over.

BRYANT: What kind of results have you observed from the combination of chemotherapeutic drugs with immunological approaches to cancer therapy?

ZIGHELBOIM: We've found that combining or integrating approaches like this can be very beneficial. For instance, experiments show that some chemotherapeutic drugs, given in a certain context, can actually facilitate the action of the immune system. Exposure of cancer cells to certain cytotoxic drugs followed by immunologic intervention leads to better results than either immunological or chemotherapeutic treatments alone. In these cases, the chemotherapy agent is actually used as a means of sensitizing or priming the cells to be destroyed by other mechanisms.

BRYANT: How do the immunological and chemotherapeutic agents interact?

ZIGHELBOIM: Certain components of the immune system suppress the immune system's response to the cancer. We call these suppressor cells. Chemotherapeutic drugs may play the role of altering those suppressor cells to allow for better activity against cancerous growth. As affected by the chemotherapeutic drug, these very same suppressor cells may actually facilitate a beneficial immune process. There is also evidence that certain cytotoxic drugs actually complement biologic molecules like interferon in ways we still don't understand. We have observed that if you use interferon with a certain chemotherapeutic drug, you will get a better response than if you used either substance on its own. All of these concepts are just now beginning to be explored; it's all still in the experimental stage.

BRYANT: Can you describe, from a scientific point of view, the field of immunology called psychoneuroimmunology?

ZIGHELBOIM: Psychoneuroimmunology says that there are major connections between the brain, the endocrine system and the immune system. Simply put, the brain affects the immune system. If we destroy a certain center in the brain, the functions of the immune system will be affected. If a person is depressed, the cells will not react as well to certain medications.

Psychoneuroimmunology is also investigating the effects of conditioning—ways in which you can condition immune responses so that, for instance, a certain stimulus will cause the immune system to react in a certain way. All sorts of research is being done in this area.

BRYANT: I would be especially interested to hear about studies which support the hypothesis that certain practices ranging from laughter to prayer can stimulate the immune system to deal more effectively with disease.

ZIGHELBOIM: Most of the scientific evidence that's been gathered suggests that a great deal of negative conditioning has been achieved. If you do certain things, you will inhibit certain immune reactions. It stands to reason that if one set of psychological factors can depress the immune system, another set of psychological factors might stimulate it. But no scientific evidence that I know of supports this idea.

There *is* evidence that under hypnosis an individual's immune reactions can be altered in response to certain stimuli, for instance. The use of techniques such as transcendental meditation and creative imagery has also been studied. There are many possibilities and avenues of research in the area of psychology. However, although several studies do support the idea of relationship between the mind and the body, they don't go as far as to say that the way your psyche is functioning directly affects the body's functions, or that there is a psychic component to every sickness. From a scientific point of view, there are relationships here, but we don't yet know how far these relationships go or how significant they are. Looking at things from a scientific perspective, we simply have no proof.

BRYANT: I've heard about a great deal of work in guided imagery, through which people are told to imagine white blood cells killing or eating up their cancer.

ZIGHELBOIM: We are currently working here at UCLA with women who have ovarian cancer. The technique we're experimenting with is called guided affective imagery. The patient is taken to a special place such as a meadow or a cave where she may meet her inner self. She's not told what will happen. The images will flow spontaneously.

Guided affective imagery and other types of imagery have a great deal of research potential, and may have a great deal of merit. At least they're attracting the interest of scientists, which is a very positive thing, I think. The difficulty with proving the value of such techniques scientifically is that there are a tremendous number of variables which must be controlled. But it can be done. It is possible.

BRYANT: What work is being done to understand the relationship between stress and human health?

ZIGHELBOIM: There are studies focusing solely on the effects of stress upon the immune system. Individuals experience different patterns of activity in reaction to stress according to their personalities. People who are very depressed or who are mourning, for instance, experience an impairment in immune processes. Maybe they get more colds or infections, or perhaps they have more accidents. It's been shown, too, that we tend to get colds or other illnesses at particular times of the year—holidays, for example, or when stressful things come up. I know several people who are particularly accident-prone whenever they're under a great deal of stress. The stress diffuses their alertness. This causes a disharmony. The accident is both a result and a reminder.

BRYANT: A way of saying, "You're not paying attention or being mindful enough." An accident or illness might also be saying, "You're not resting or relaxing enough."

ZIGHELBOIM: That may be it. Behind it all is the fact that there are deep connections and interplay among the physical and psychological systems within and around us.

Ultimately, there is nothing that can be strictly labeled "central nervous system" or "immune system." There are no compartments. You can't say that the appendix belongs just to the immune system, or that the pituitary gland belongs only to the endocrine system. It's all interdependent. It's all happening together. It's simply a totality.

We recognize an integrating principle or force that is affected by all these very sophisticated systems within the body. But in terms of scientific research, we haven't reached the point where we can say that if you have a certain type of attitude, or if you visualize certain things in a certain way, you'll be able to cure your disease.

BRYANT: Can you talk more about the work being done at UCLA in the field of psychoneuroimmunology?

ZIGHELBOIM: The underlying premise of the work is simply that if one mental state can depress your immune system, another mental state can stimulate it. Attitude somehow does reflect upon physiology. The idea behind our work with patients who have ovarian cancer is to find out whether imagery influences a certain function. Of course, we may mistakenly choose to study the wrong function. We're just beginning to look into that domain. Once we get some results, and some understanding, then we have a foundation from which to build.

BRYANT: How has your own process of finding you had cancer, and working with your cancer, affected your view of medicine?

ZIGHELBOIM: Living with the realization that I had cancer, I began to feel a new attraction to certain things, an awareness of new connections. I began to see that health has to be affected by what we do and how we live. I became more aware of what I was eating and why I was eating. I became more conscious of my dreams and feelings and intuitions. Basically, I became more attuned to my own inner process.

BRYANT: Can you talk about how these breakthroughs affected your personal and professional life?

ZIGHELBOIM: My life here at the medical center was always so busy. I had things to do in the lab, with patients or at home. I always had things to read and write and plan. There was no time, really, to be in touch with the inner level. The moment I stopped doing things and started moving slower and reminding myself, "You don't have to read anything now, you can just sit," I began to sense certain things for the first time, and I had new perceptions and ideas. I began to appreciate the richness of the inner life — images and feelings. I began to get in touch with important dream images which I hadn't been paying attention to. All of these things had been going on before, but I wasn't aware of them. They were just not part of me. Attuning to my inner process allowed and created the time and space to be with my inner self. I found an incredible richness of insight and understanding and intuition — all kinds of things which can't be appreciated when a busy-busy level of activity and thoughts overshadows these areas.

BRYANT: What are some of the results of this attunement in your life?

ZIGHELBOIM: Most important for me is that I've begun to experience a congruence, or unification, in all that I do. Part of my struggle is to break the partitions between work life, family life and spiritual life. My process of growing awareness and inner vision is part of the same process that is expressed through my research. I've become aware of how wisdom and intuition complement knowledge gained from more rational or logical ways of knowing.

BRYANT: How have your colleagues reacted to what might be interpreted as a rejection of science?

ZIGHELBOIM: I haven't rejected science. I teach immunology to medical students. I speak the scientific language. My ability to bridge what might be seen as two worlds has actually helped me enormously in putting forward what I need to express. My colleagues have been receptive. I've found that there is fertile ground within the system to allow for expansion and new possibilities. The field of psychoneuroimmunology is witness to that.

BRYANT: Do you see psychoneuroimmunology as a link between Oriental and Occidental medical systems?

ZIGHELBOIM: I feel more and more that when we move into a deeper state of attunement with the deeper aspects of ourselves, we can tap into wisdom that is universal. It's not mine; it's not yours or theirs; it's ours. What happens then is that we begin to draw from a common source. Some call it a collective unconscious. Others call it something else. I don't know what to call it, but I see it as a sort of data base that we learn to enter. It's a vast data base with a lot of information and wisdom. If we learn how to access the right program, we can know and do a lot of things. That's one way to put it. It's not mysterious.

It may very well be that polarization between Eastern and Western systems of thought and medicine has been essential for the developmental process. Western science has made awesome strides, and is a tremendous wealth in itself. The ancient Oriental sciences have also made tremendous discoveries over thousands of years. Perhaps in this generation, we'll begin to explore and experience the rich benefits of blending these two systems.

Many of us are beginning to wake up to this, bringing forward alternatives that blend rather than discount, that integrate rather than substitute, and that encompass rather than exclude. I feel a great richness when I'm working with a patient, aware that I have access to all these resources. I can draw upon pharmacology, hematology, oncology, psychology, immunology, spirituality and so on. It's an enormous pool of resources which can be brought forward. It contrasts with the polarized, limited place which I experienced before. But I do feel that my initiation process within the tradition of Western science was essential, for grounding and for balance.

BRYANT: It seems clear that in your life cancer has been a teacher.

ZIGHELBOIM: It's been one of the best things that ever happened to me in terms of how it opened me, and what I've experienced from that. I know that I may have been opened to these things in other ways, but it's unlikely that it would have happened so soon.

BRYANT: Can you talk about the Healing the Self conferences you've initiated? How are you expressing your philosophy? What are you learning as you work?

ZIGHELBOIM: Through my work, I've come to recognize the importance of emotional and spiritual nourishment for optimum health. Of course, we all know that we need to eat well, but the importance of other nourishing factors is less evident. We need a continuous supply of emotional and spiritual nourishment to maintain balance. The body needs to be stroked and touched, which does not happen enough. And it needs to be nourished spiritually. This can happen physically or otherwise. Somewhere in our development, this nourishment becomes disturbed and diminished as a result of many factors, which may or may not be measurable.

I perceive that at the root of illness, there is an isolation, a detachment from nourishment—as much psychological and spiritual as physical.

Many of us are living in a malnourished psycho-spiritual state. And the lack of attunement to these needs, with no satisfaction of these needs, leads to a general depletion which fosters or could foster the development of disease.

The root of health, then, is found in seeking and attaining nourishment. There are many ways to do it.

BRYANT: Do you think that a person who is well nourished psychologically and spiritually is less susceptible to illness and more able to deal with stress?

ZIGHELBOIM: I think that an individual who is well nourished and well attended is more able to take conditions which are stressful and respond to them effectively, without feeling burdened or distressed by them. An individual who is depleted and alienated is less capable of responding, because the nourishment of love and warmth, which the body needs, is unavailable.

I see this as happening parallel to the way it happens on a physical level. Malnourishment on the organic level creates an environment which fosters the development of illness, because the body is debilitated. We know that malnutrition is a conditioning factor for illness, not a specific illness. Many different illnesses are simply more likely to occur in a malnourished population. So we need to pay more attention to this.

BRYANT: What do you see as being the most important factor in the nourishing process? Family? Community?

ZIGHELBOIM: Family and community have something to do with it, but fundamentally, I see it as something which begins with the individual, and then moves from there to the family, and then the community. So the healing and the satisfaction of these needs is an individual process. When the individual accepts his or her vulnerability and nourishes and provides for herself or himself, compassion is being practiced. This compassion for self then develops and extends to others. Personal relationships begin to come into the potential for healing. This process is reflected out to the family, then to society.

BRYANT: But basically, you're saying that it has to start with the individual.

ZIGHELBOIM: Yes. If you're married, for instance, you simply start to move in the direction which provides you with the most nourishment. This creates the potential for your partner to move toward whatever is most nourishing for her or him. As two people move, the potential is created for others surrounding them to move.

The moment you recognize your own vulnerability and your own need for nourishment, the healing begins. But one person must make the decision, and begin the work. You can't wait for everyone else around you to do it.

BRYANT: So personal vulnerability and our basic need for nourishment are fundamental aspects of your work during Healing the Self conferences.

ZIGHELBOIM: Yes, I present these ideas to people as they become clear and take shape in my own mind. I'm also working to bring forth the resources of nourishment for myself and for those who surround me, including my patients and others who are simply attracted to what I say.

BRYANT: Is it sometimes difficult to reconcile such a theory with your identity as a scientist?

ZIGHELBOIM: If we waited for everything to be proven before believing, nothing would ever be discovered—or proven, for that matter. Until we know these scientific facts, what are we to do? Are we to wait? Are we to stop exploring and presenting that which we see as valuable? Or do we present these ideas and allow people to come to their own conclusions based on their own experiences?

I'm looking into ways of exploring my own findings—the things I know through intuition and my own experience—according to scientific methodology. I'm involved in an ongoing effort to validate these ideas according to the resources and technology available to us in the 1990s.

BRYANT: With regard to the Healing the Self conferences, what exactly are your goals?

ZIGHELBOIM: The conferences offer people a chance to expand their awareness and perspectives—to go inside, to explore levels we might ordinarily never get to in our ordinary lives. The purpose of the conference is to facilitate healing.

BRYANT: How do you define healing?

ZIGHELBOIM: First, it doesn't necessarily mean the reconstitution of physical health. Healing is the process of creating balance and harmony through opening to deeper levels of reality and experience. Normally, we may be unaware of this place within. Our goal is movement toward that harmonious balance, whether one has come to help deal with physical illness, emotional conflict, or a work-related disturbance.

The workshop is also an opportunity for people to live in an environment where they can focus totally and concentrate on what really interests them. They can live and communicate and share with other human beings in new ways which reveal new possibilities in human relationships. It's a highly nourishing environment. There are no pressures, no expectations, no responsibilities. People have an opportunity to do absolutely anything they want to do, perhaps for the first time in their lives. Of course, there are difficulties related to being free of responsibilities and expectations. We explore those challenges.

BRYANT: Earlier you mentioned that when you became more aware of your own inner process, you became aware of images from your dreams. Do you focus on dreams during Healing the Self?

ZIGHELBOIM: A lot of the work involves looking into messages and information that come from the unconscious, through dreams, spontaneous images or insights. This gives people an opportunity to experience altered states of consciousness so that they can feel more, understand more, and sense more. The work helps people to broaden their horizons as to who they are, and to see what the experiences that they are involved with represent. The idea is to receive a direct sense through first-hand experience of their capacities, their options, and their resources when confronted with illness or other potentially threatening situations.

So they come out, hopefully, with a deeper appreciation of life and the life forces that they're involved with, a deeper understanding of their capacities to balance and to heal, perhaps a heightened sense of their potential, and most important, with resources and techniques to go on exploring and journeying and living more fully.

BRYANT: During the week of the conference, what kind of schedule do you follow?

ZIGHELBOIM: Daily, we start with a collective meditation at around 6 A.M. That goes on for about forty-five minutes. Then we have dreamwork from about 7 A.M. to 8 or 8:30 A.M. The dreamwork is more than intellectual analysis; it's really about feeling into the dream. That is, we try to keep ourselves open to the feeling of what the dream is trying to reveal. We also look at the context of the dream, the images themselves, and the forces in the dream. But we stress the feeling.

After a group session in the morning, we have the afternoons completely free. During our night session, we explore different areas of experience. Sometimes we use music; sometimes we use body movement; other times we use meditation; or we might use creative imagery.

We try to perceive and enter experiences in new ways, to broaden our perspective of what reality is, and to realize that we function in relative, subjective reality. From our own individual perspective, our reality is the only reality. But for others, it's not. This breaks down the sense of doom, because something that seems hopeless from one perspective may have a completely different configuration when we expand into another area of our psyche — another perspective.

BRYANT: So participants are introduced to seeing the world and themselves through expanded dimensions of the psyche. What kind of effect does this have on people?

ZIGHELBOIM: One very important part of the workshop is the recognition of our sacredness — the realization that we are, all of us, holy beings. When we try to relate to one another on that level, we see a tremendous change in the way most people perceive themselves and the people they live, work and play with. Everyday reality is seen from a totally different vantage point. And yet we maintain the consciousness that ordinary awareness is also real.

The idea is not to escape it and go off into some kind of ethereal level, but to appreciate that there is more. Simply, we're brought to the realization that the more potential we can encompass, the more capacities we can embody. Working from a limited perspective, we can only do and be what that particular perspective is capable of seeing and being. But we can go beyond that. We can acquire capacities, resources and potentials which require our moving past the areas that we were once confined to by our own limited self-perceptions. It's a transforming event.

BRYANT: What you're saying here seems consistent with what you said earlier about the immune system. Perhaps certain levels of consciousness are more able to affect our physical health than others. Perhaps the stimulation of new types of thinking, new images and ideas about ourselves, can also stimulate the immune system's potential.

ZIGHELBOIM: Actually, multipersonality research is beginning to reveal that the state of the mind and the state of the brain are indeed related to the way the immune system responds to the brain. Different signals may be delivered from the brain centers and through the mind to the immune system and the endocrine system, depending upon one's physical and mental state. Perhaps when you alter your state, when you heighten your awareness to connect with the universal "healer energy" inside of you, your immune system receives a signal which encourages recovery or healing. Maybe when you're connected with an aspect of victimization, or feel highly dependent or incapable, the cues and the stimuli to the immune system reflect that, and it responds appropriately.

BRYANT: You've come a ways here from the language of medical science.

ZIGHELBOIM: Perhaps I've strayed from scientific language, but really none of this is mysterious or esoteric or out of this world. I think we're talking about the acquisition and expression of human potential, which is quite vast.

The resources I've been talking about, whether you want to call them psychoneuroimmunology or "healing energy" or "spirit," are all just part of the human capacity. It may all be contained in what we are as part of our heritage—part of our collective wisdom. I believe that all of this knowledge and ability is contained within us as part of the incredible resources which we all have, but which have not come to full expression.

BRYANT: What are the catalysts you see as being needed in order to allow and encourage the allopathic medical system to open up more, and to better respond to psychological and other factors affecting patients' health?

ZIGHELBOIM: It has already begun to open up, to an extent. There is certainly an awakening, among physicians and within society, of the importance of the potential of mind, the interaction between mind and body, the role of that interaction in the physiology of the individual, and the importance of psychosocial factors in illness. Also, I think growing numbers of doctors are beginning to appreciate that medicine which is limited to mechanics and technology is simply not complete.

In general, I'd say that dissatisfaction with medical services comes not only from patients, but also from doctors themselves. I think all of this is leading toward more emphasis on the psychological and human aspects of support, with patients being more involved in their own care and management.

BRYANT: What do you see as some of the practical effects of these changes?

ZIGHELBOIM: As awareness grows, some of these elements begin to be included in medical school curriculum. And as doctors learn more about these areas, they make use of them in their practices and in their nonprofessional lives.

Of course, part of the pressure for such changes comes from the patients themselves. As they voice their concerns, the medical community will have to respond more broadly with practical solutions.

BRYANT: Although you're describing an ongoing change in very positive terms, some of the ideas we've discussed here may also be seen as a threat to scientific medical practice.

ZIGHELBOIM: Any issue which threatens a belief system or way of perceiving something will cause resistance. But I've learned that the greater the resistance, the more important is the issue for the person who is resisting it. Something that threatens you will always be related to some critical issues in your life. You won't take any interest in something that isn't an important issue for you. The response of active rejection or suppression is usually linked with feeling threatened. The rejection functions to help you avoid dealing with some issue which is actually rather important, but which is frightening, angering, or simply inconvenient. It may take weeks or months or years to really deal with it. No matter how valuable the information, it may simply be too demanding.

BRYANT: And on an individual level?

ZIGHELBOIM: Individually, we have to deal with threats to personal beliefs, personal perspectives, our ideals, the way we conduct our lives and do things. We don't want to change and look into those things if we don't have to. We're greatly devoted to the status quo.

BRYANT: Do you think that this is related somehow to the busy-ness of our lives—the fact that we simply don't take the time to know ourselves as well and as deeply as we could?

ZIGHELBOIM: Yes. Often we find ourselves living in ways that do not honor or appreciate who we are in our multiple aspects. We live in ways that ignore many of our inner resources. We act and react, responding to old patterns. And if we don't know the forces of the psyche that move through us, we'll be continually vul-nerable. So our buttons get pushed. We react without understand-ing. We reject ideas. We're threatened, often as a result of a divorce between our rational minds, our daily activities, and many areas of our inner life. We simply don't recognize how a particular issue which we see as threatening may be the key to increased under-standing of self and others. We don't recognize its importance in our life.

BRYANT: How do you think that the awareness you're talking about will contribute to advances in medicine, specifically cancer medicine? How do you envision the cancer medicine of the fu-ture?

ZIGHELBOIM: I think that the whole perspective on cancer is going to open up. We'll see a much broader approach to the can-cer patient. Psychospiritual and psychosocial points of view will play greater roles. We'll see movement away from the aggressive therapies, toward the biological therapies.

BRYANT: What will the results of this movement be?

ZIGHELBOIM: The immunological approach is less militaris-tic. We may actually find drugs which will make cells mature and normalize their function. I also foresee that surgery, radiation and chemotherapy will become archaic in the near future. We won't be using them, or we'll be using them much less.

BRYANT: What about prevention of cancer?

ZIGHELBOIM: That, to me, is a much larger undertaking. I don't know how ready we are, as a society, to conceive of it. It may just be that the way of life we're developing is part of what we'll have to change. But I don't see us making great leaps in that area, at least right now. People in general are terrified of change.

BRYANT: You see people as preferring to live with the risk of getting cancer rather than making the necessary personal and so-cietal changes to prevent it?

ZIGHELBOIM: You're talking about making big changes, which is fearful, and no one can guarantee that if we make changes, cancer will go away. I think it's a matter of evolution, and I think our motivations for many of the changes we may have to make will have to go beyond just avoiding cancer.

BRYANT: You seem to have come full circle from your work as an immunologist and physician to some of the most basic aspects of medicine—compassion and nourishment among them.

ZIGHELBOIM: It's a return to basics, but one which doesn't throw technological developments out the window. The ideal is a blending, and an integration. We should strive for an appreciation of the fundamental psychological and spiritual aspects of the human being. We should strive to go beyond the limitations set by purely mechanical approaches to medicine. At the same time, we should recognize what these approaches have to offer. When and if some of our methods stop offering important benefits, or when there are new and better approaches which can be substituted for them, then we'll let the outmoded ways go.

Cancer As Teacher

DWIGHT McKEE, M.D.

Dr. Dwight McKee's path as a medical doctor has taken him from standard allopathic medical training to collaboration with explorers on the forefront of medical research. Working in modalities ranging from chemotherapy to nutrition to metabolic therapies and transformational psychological approaches, Dr. McKee has been active in the field of cancer research and treatment since 1975, and has served as private physician to the XVI Gyalwa Karmapa. Having taught extensively throughout the U.S., Dr. McKee is currently enrolled as a medical resident. He will resume medical practice as an oncologist in 1994.

INTRODUCTION

Dr. Dwight McKee was one of the first medical professionals I interviewed in researching cancer for this book. His work with standard allopathic treatments as well as with nonconventional medical practices gives him a broad perspective on cancer and the cancer-care community. He offered me an invaluable introduction to medical trends and terminology, preparing me to enter new areas of discussion with greater familiarity and ease.

Dr. McKee also introduced me to several historical characters whose contributions to medical practice seem relevant to today's world. One such character was Dr. Semmelweiss, whose work preceded Pasteur's discovery of bacteria. Dr. Semmelweiss was in charge of a ward at the Vienna women's hospital at a time when a woman who gave birth in a hospital had a fifty-fifty chance of surviving childbed fever. Semmelweiss recognized a dangerous association between doctors' doing autopsies and then delivering babies immediately afterward. When he began washing his hands between the morgue and the delivery room, he found that his patients stopped dying of childbed fever. Unable to impress upon his colleagues the importance of this sanitary measure, Dr. Semmelweiss ended up standing guard on his ward, refusing to admit any doctor who hadn't washed his hands. The incidence of childbed fever on his ward dropped dramatically, but his theory was never accepted during his lifetime. In order for doctors to have admitted that Dr. Semmelweiss was right, they would have had to admit to poor medical practice on their own part.

Dr. McKee tells this story as an aid to "getting past the fear" of opening up to new as well as ancient methods of medical practice which may lead to new perspectives and important advances in the science of healing.

During a time of increasing specialization by medical professionals, Dr. McKee is able to speak clearly and authoritatively about many of the world's medical systems, while communicating the commonality of these systems. He stresses the shared motivation of all healers to ease suffering, and functions as a catalyst for intercultural and interdisciplinary exchange.

DIALOGUE

BRYANT: You've had a great deal of experience working on the development and application of various approaches to cancer treatment. What do you see as being our greatest medical problem today?

McKEE: From my perspective, the most basic problem seems to be that we're focusing far more on disease care than on health care. In fact, we're spending a good ten percent of the gross national product on disease care alone. We've totally ignored preventive medicine. Instead of helping people to stay healthy, we focus our energy on finding cures for illnesses that have already developed dramatic symptoms. Our medical system simply does not prepare us to deal with the general, free-floating feeling of unwellness which offers people the greatest problem today.

BRYANT: The syndrome you're describing sounds like what I call "pre-disease."

McKEE: Yes. The most common symptom of "pre-disease," a run-down, blah feeling, doesn't usually show up on blood tests or EKGs or x-rays. People experiencing these symptoms deserve treatment, but they're cheated by our medical system, which seems to say, "We aren't interested in helping you unless you're gravely ill." Modern, western M.D.s have been trained to treat only full-blown diseases. Far too often, when a patient comes in feeling "not right," he or she is told, "You're fine." The M.D. might write a prescription for a tranquilizer or send the patient to see a psychiatrist. But we're finding that psychosomatic complaints are related to physical causes like stress, lack of exercise, or poor nutrition.

If we were truly interested in maintaining health, we would intervene when a patient first complains. We would find out about stress patterns, work and family situations, diet and exercise habits, how much coffee, alcohol, tobacco and other drugs are consumed. We would encourage lifestyle changes and basic health awareness, and see if these changes lead to an alteration of patients' complaints. In general, we would strive to strengthen the patient so that full-blown diseases don't get a chance to develop.

BRYANT: Do you feel that making these lifestyle changes and adopting more healthy habits can actually prevent diseases as serious as cancer?

McKEE: It's not easy to say whether cancer can be prevented through lifestyle changes, but preventive medicine is certainly worth a lot more attention than it is currently given.

When we look into the case histories of cancer patients, it's common to find that these people have been going to doctors for three years or so with general complaints. They've been told, "There's nothing wrong with you," because doctors could find nothing wrong through physical examination or the usual battery of tests. Our tendency not to look beyond acute pathology ignores the presence of factors that weaken health, and negates our ability to prevent disease. It's dangerous, because people never learn to build up their resistance to disease.

BRYANT: What kind of preventive measures do you recommend that people take to help them stay or become physically balanced?

McKEE: It's extremely important to avoid excesses of all drugs, including tobacco, alcohol and coffee. These substances create an imbalance, and in response, the body expends a great deal of energy in attempting to restore that balance. But the best preventive measures are simply the practices which contribute to good health: eating a varied diet of wholesome food, exercising, being in touch with emotions, being creative, doing the things that make you happy — things you really want to do.

All aspects of one's lifestyle contribute toward balance or imbalance, and I believe that a balanced life promotes a balanced body. Balance involves a person's entire being, including his or her attitudes.

BRYANT: How much of a role do you think attitude plays in our ability to prevent and even treat cancer?

McKEE: To my mind, attitude determines the entire direction of cancer research and treatment, on both individual and community levels.

When people are confronted with cancer, the ones who tend to do well are generally those who stop and take a look at their lives — those who are willing to evaluate what is and what isn't important to them. They're the ones who are sincerely willing to change many of their own patterns. They'll stop smoking; they're willing to change their diets or the way they relate to their families and friends. They are strong enough and flexible enough to drop away from many of the old patterns of living associated with the cancer-producing physiology.

On the other hand, people who rigidly hold on to their old ways of being and simply invoke the doctor to give them drugs or radiation to obliterate the "enemy" that's invaded their bodies typically don't do well.

It is essential that as individuals we look at personal patterns and evaluate them. This allows us to work with and change the things that appear to have a negative effect on our emotions or on other aspects of our lives.

BRYANT: But even great changes in attitude and lifestyle might not be enough if a cancer is caused by factors which we don't have much control over.

McKEE: Yes, exactly—including environmental hazards and a number of other problems. Individuals aren't living in a vacuum. We are all affected by societal conditions and the energies surrounding them. Still, it makes sense to invoke what we do know about personal health care, even knowing that working toward our own personal well-being may simply not be enough.

BRYANT: A great many people are taking more responsibility for their own health by turning to health practitioners who encourage their active participation. There are chiropractors who deal with nutrition, naturopathic physicians and others who deal with many aspects of preventive medicine, including nutrition, exercise and stress control. Plus, more and more chemotherapists, radiologists and surgeons are advocating dietary modifications or other forms of adjunctive therapy to complement their treatment.

McKEE: Yes, this is a very fortunate thing. Increasing networks of personal computers, the development of "expert" software systems, marketing of laboratory diagnostic tests directly to the consumer, and a renaissance in the personal use of nutrition, herbology and homeopathy are some of the emerging forces which may radically transform the health-care field over the next decade.

BRYANT: Do you think this will help doctors to overcome what seems like a tremendous chasm between conventional modern practice and holistic medicine?

McKEE: Up till now, polarization between the emerging American Holistic Medical Association and the vastly powerful AMA (American Medical Association) has been extremely counterproductive. In 1982, the AMA took away the AHMA's ability to grant credits for an important category of continuing education because the Holistic Association doesn't maintain a full-time, paid committee on continuing education. As if the American Holistic Medical Association could afford such a thing!

Actions like this just widen the gap. Only in 1986 did we begin to see signs of reconciliation and broader mutual acceptance.

Today, more doctors who are personally dissatisfied with their medical practices, and others who simply want more dialogue with the holistic medical community, are joining the American Holistic Medical Association. This represents a growing number of physicians who are picking up on and using holistic methods and attitudes. So things are changing, little by little.

BRYANT: Where do you think the impetus for change is coming from?

McKEE: A great deal of the pressure comes from the patient, but change is also coming from the doctors themselves. Today, many doctors are jogging or running for their own health, and they enjoy treating fellow runners. Doctors are discovering how nutrition can make drastic differences in their own lives. As a result, they pay attention to their patients' nutrition.

Then we have doctors who take care of themselves through diet and excercise for instance, while still practicing very conventional medicine in terms of the diagnosis and treatment of their patients. But even practicing conventionally, they are certainly a far cry from the overweight, heavy smoker who advises his patients to stop smoking and to lose weight.

BRYANT: Generally, what are some ways of making orthodox medical practice more effective?

McKEE: I think we should change the criteria by which students are selected for medical school. Today, the schools select for a highly focused, intense left-brain type person, with a tendency toward linear thinking and logical analysis. Often, due to the rigors of academic competition, these students do little else but study. The result is that they don't have a chance to develop effective interpersonal communication skills. So we produce doctors who don't communicate well with their patients, or who are focused completely on technology or some other aspect of medicine which is divorced from human relationships.

But I see the beginnings of a positive trend in this area as well. A good number of studies have been conducted on aspects of medical training, with the aim of finding out how to get a more well-rounded type of person into medicine, and more women into medicine. That certainly is going to bring about some balance.

BRYANT: We spoke a bit earlier about the importance of the patient's attitude in the healing process. But what about the doctor's attitude?

McKEE: Physicians who believe in what they're doing will always have better results than those who simply follow procedures they've been taught. I believe that the physician's attitude can actually affect the patient's immune response.

BRYANT: I know that when I was a kid, the doctor's bedside manner had a tremendous effect on my outlook. Can you can talk more about how the immune system is related to the mind?

McKEE: Psychoneuroimmunology is an entire field of study. The link between the mind and the immune system has been shown in many studies with animals. For instance, monkeys have been exposed to a substance which increases or decreases their white blood cell count; at the same time, they're exposed to a specific odor. Later, when exposed only to the odor, they have had the same white blood cell response! This shows that the immune system can be conditioned and affected by many factors. That's just a simple demonstration of the immune system's relationship to the mind. It's a very fertile field of research right now.

BRYANT: Can you describe the effects of meditation and other contemplative activities which reduce stress and tension? Biophysically or biochemically, what actually takes place?

McKEE: Stress stimulates the sympathetic nervous system, activating our adrenal glands, which secrete adrenalin and prepare us for confrontation or for "flight" away from the threat. Meditation and other contemplative activities have just the opposite effect, quieting the activity of the sympathetic nervous system. At the same time, contemplative activites tend to enhance the activity of the *para*sympathetic nervous system, which supports the digestive system as well as the immune system. Regular practice of both meditation and visualization has been shown to help cancer patients increase the number of lymphocytes available to them, and it may also be of benefit as a preventive measure.

BRYANT: Do you feel that the practice of compassion by medical professionals, family members and others involved in enhancing patients' well-being might have similar soothing and healing effects?

McKEE: I think that exposure to love or compassion helps to balance the energy field of the patient. It helps to quiet the nervous system and to stop the secretion of fear-stimulated adrenalin. This is important because fear can raise physiological havoc. Fear suppresses the immune system, and is certainly one of the most deadly aspects of cancer.

BRYANT: Over the phone recently, you mentioned having lost a cancer patient who came through a great deal of fear and underwent dramatic psychological growth during treatment. Can you talk about some of the lessons you learned during your work with her?

McKEE: Lynda was a 19-year-old with lymphoblastic lymphoma. She was facing a difficult period of her life, and had witnessed the death of several family members who had gone through chemotherapy treatments unsuccessfully. She was afraid of her disease, but she was also afraid of living. She felt trapped.

We worked with dreams, did family therapy, visualization, and a great deal of voice dialogue—a means of exploring the psyche through a combination of Jungian work, transactional analysis, Gestalt, psychodrama, and psycho-synthesis. We also used radiation, limited chemotherapy, nutrition and other modes of treatment.

I've always learned from my patients on a personal level. Some patients have helped to guide me toward study; others have helped me by giving my practice a new emphasis. Lynda did both. Although she died, she grew in many beautiful ways during her illness. She grew stronger, more self-aware, more hopeful, more accepting, more communicative. Lynda showed me all the elements that need to be brought together in dealing with a person who is ill. In her case, the process of stabilizing her physical condition was secondary—a means of buying time for her to explore herself, to understand the meaning of her illness and the shifts she needed to make in order to become psychologically whole. Becoming psychologically whole does not always mean physical recovery. She didn't recover physically.

My experience with Lynda introduced me to a lot of the latest technology being used in cancer treatment. Partly as a result, I decided to go back into residency in oncology so as to better study the new technology.

BRYANT: Do you still feel a commitment to working with experimental methods, and to your work as a communicator?

McKEE: Absolutely. I see myself primarily as an integrator— someone with a broad view of what methods are available and how they can be most effectively combined. We need to develop systems which can deal with the psyche, and we need access to the technology which can stabilize physical symptoms. We need to learn how to use modern technology more flexibly. I want to become much more familiar with technological innovations and trends so that I can better contribute to the research that tells us how it can all be combined.

BRYANT: The hospice movement is working to improve the psychological and spiritual state of cancer patients facing death, but dealing with death and dying is still far from being a medical priority.

McKEE: We have a long way to go.

BRYANT: At this point, what do you see as being some of the strong points or advantages of conventional cancer treatments?

McKEE: As a result of early diagnosis and treatment, better surgical techniques, and a better understanding of the toxicity of chemotherapy drugs, conventional cancer medicine is succeeding at helping people to live for five years or more after diagnosis. But one of the most serious problems we face when looking at those five-year success stories is that it is extremely misleading to consider people who live for five years beyond diagnosis to be "cured."

In a study published in *The New England Journal of Medicine* in May of 1986, Dr. John Bailar—formerly of the National Cancer Institute and now of the Harvard Department of Public Health— points out that the yearly death rates from cancer have steadily risen in spite of improved "five-year survival" statistics.

BRYANT: What do you see as being a solution?

McKEE: In general, I think we have to orient ourselves to a more receptive approach to healing. Attacking a tumor as if it were an enemy is just one way of looking at cancer. We can also choose to approach cancer as a problem due to environmental and personal factors—a problem that can teach us something.

Instead of working with the receptive, responsive energies of cooperative problem-solving, we have favored the aggressive, polarizing energies. Toxic waste dumps, nuclear pollution, pesticides in our food chain, the overprocessing of our food so that it is stripped of vital nutrients, and widespread war are all manifestations of this aggressive energy gone unchecked. Our approach to cancer reflects a military approach to medicine. Poison the tumor. Kill the tumor. I'm sure this language is familiar to you. In fact, all the agents of modern cancer therapy are referred to as an "armamentarium."

BRYANT: But it seems appropriate to use a military model in fighting cancer. After all, isn't it true that within the body itself, cancer cells actually "invade" the body in a way that could be considered militaristic?

McKEE: The way we perceive and understand what happens in the body has a geat deal to do with a whole package of assumptions and perceptions that we're not even aware of, because we're brought up with them. In science, the way we see things has a great deal to do with the minds of the people developing the theories. There are many different ways of seeing the same set of sequences and events. Take the natural law of "kill or be killed — survival of the fittest." We focus on the competitive aspects of survival, but instead we could look at the struggle for survival as a cooperative system engineered to effect the "greatest good for all." Ultimately, one's perspective depends very much on one's own mindset and mental filter. We can always choose to see things differently and work with them in new, positive and more productive ways.

BRYANT: You're describing a basic philosophical problem: we're unable to recognize the framework which shapes our thoughts because our thoughts themselves are limited by that framework.

McKEE: Yes. We only talk about "killer cells" in the immune system because the medical model is steeped in that militaristic way of seeing things. As we see cooperative action replacing competitive action, our ways of seeing and judging most phenomena will have changed and will continue to change.

BRYANT: But when you're sick, it's very hard to see illness as a learning experience, for instance. Many of us tend to see our bodies as if they were machines whose mechanisms have somehow run amok. We take on a sort of macho, defensive attitude: sickness is a sign of weakness. "Who, me? I'm not sick. This is just a temporary breakdown. I'm perfectly healthy. Strong as a bull."

McKEE: You call that type of attitude "macho," and it's true that the attitude you're describing is identified with male ego, whether it's found in a man or a woman. It's a confrontational attitude toward disease, and it goes along with our desire to.kill off a disease, not listen to it. What I'm trying to get across is that it's not the only attitude, or the best attitude.

John Wayne was a perfect example of someone who chose the macho style of dealing with illness. He was "cured" of cancer when his lung was removed in surgery. He raised enormous sums of money for the American Cancer Society with his "I beat the big C" campaign, and then died ten years later of a recurrence of the lung

cancer. Given his lifestyle and inflexibility, this was totally predictable.

Incidentally, having survived more than five years after treatment,
Wayne persists in the statistics as a cure, along with millions of
others who have died of recurring cancer.

BRYANT: So he was really living on what we call "false hope."

McKEE: It's interesting that you use that expression. Actually,
"false hope" is the most frequent accusation used by the medical
establishment toward alternative practitioners. But consider this:
a sixty-year-old gentleman gets cancer of the colon. He's operated
upon, and they say, "We got it all." That patient then says, "Great.
I've been cured." So he goes right back to his old ways of living,
with no changes, no awareness that maybe he should take a look
at the patterns that contributed to his getting cancer in the first
place. He thinks he's simply been cured, once and for all. Well,
it's very likely that two years later, the cancer will be in his liver
or recurrent in his abdomen.

The doctors say, "It's a kindness to let the man think he's cured,
because then he'll be able to enjoy two good years." They don't
know what else to do. In other cases, doctors are sincere in believing that they have cured such a patient. They don't see him enter
a different hospital with jaundice two years later, when the cancer
has recurred in his liver.

In thousands of such cases, a lot of false hope is generated in
the orthodox treatment of cancer through surgery. However, the
opposite may also be the case. For instance, a colon tumor has
penetrated the colon wall at the time of surgical removal. Some
surgeons who believe in "telling it like it is" will tell the patient
that based on statistics, the cancer is sure to come back. Without
being able to offer the patient strategies for changing his patterns,
the doctor's pronouncement may instill a great deal of fear and
a sense of hopelessness, which may contribute to the fulfillment
of the doctor's prognosis.

BRYANT: In neither case is the patient encouraged to make important lifestyle changes.

McKEE: Right. Cancer has an enormous potential to act as a catalyst for personal growth. It is almost always a major turning point
in people's lives.

When the threat of disease and death is presented honestly to
people, many start to think about what is really important to them.
A large number of recovered cancer patients claim to perceive their

illness as a kind of ally which opened up a new way of life to them. Some die after having the opportunity to sincerely reevaluate their lives and make significant life changes.

When used alone, conventional cancer treatment—even the best of it—is often just a means of getting rid of a tumor for five years. After that, the chances of a recurrence are greatly heightened. So a doctor's well-meaning optimism may actually undermine the patient's potential ability to make some changes that could contribute to actually preventing a recurrence. More and more people are becoming aware of this, and are taking preventive steps. Other people, who put their blind trust in what doctors tell them, are victimized by that trust.

BRYANT: I recently read an article which suggested that people today are suffering from deficient immune systems. The author seemed to be blaming everything from AIDS to cancer and herpes on inherent deficiencies in our biological make-up. Can you comment on this?

McKEE: I don't think there's anything inherently wrong with the immune system. I do think there is something inherently wrong with the way we're living on this planet. I think that one of the manifestations of this can be seen in a free-floating feeling of unwellness that is becoming increasingly common. In many cases, there's a direct connection between that unwellness and the overgrowth of a yeast called *Candida albicans.*

Candida overgrowth may make people more prone to disorders of the immune system, allergies, cancer and infectious diseases. Right now it's practically an epidemic, affecting an immense number of people who don't even know they have this imbalance within their bodies.

BRYANT: Do you see this yeast overgrowth as being caused by some aspect of modern living?

McKEE: Yes. Candida overgrowth is often stimulated by the overuse of broad-spectrum antibiotics. These antibiotics kill off not only disease-causing bacteria, but also useful, beneficial bacteria which help keep normally present yeast populations in check. Meanwhile, the primary food of yeast is sugar, and people in the U.S. eat one hundred fifty pounds of refined sugar per person, yearly, in a number of forms. This overfeeding causes the yeast to grow beyond its ecological niche. The result is an overgrowth of yeast, which represents a chronic stress on the immune system. It can cause a whole spectrum of problems, from simple, minor annoyances to symptoms which are totally incapacitating.

Clinical Candida overgrowth is commonly seen in cancer patients. Most oncologists assume this means that the immune system is depressed because of the cancer. But it may well be the reverse—the immune system may be weakened by the overgrowth of Candida, allowing cancer to develop, which then further weakens the immune system and allows the Candida to show up more obviously. I suspect that a chronic overgrowth of yeast makes a person much more susceptible to cancer, because the immune system is weakened by the constant stress involved in fighting back the yeast population.

BRYANT: What are the symptoms of Candida?

McKEE: Chronic fatigue, lethargy, difficulty concentrating, poor memory, depression and anxiety are the most common symptoms. There can be intestinal problems; irritable bowel syndrome is often related to it. Premenstrual tension in women is often related to it. Bloating after meals is another common symptom. People with Candida are also more susceptible to everything from flus and minor infections to cancer and AIDS.

BRYANT: Is it contagious?

McKEE: It may be passable between people, but Candida is primarily a harmless, normal organism. Everyone has it, and it overgrows when the immune system is compromised. We find Candida in people with AIDS, in people who have been immuno-suppressed for transplants, in cancer patients undergoing chemotherapy.

BRYANT: What happens in the body to encourage the development of cancer once the immune system becomes compromised because of the Candida?

McKEE: It is pretty well accepted theory that we all develop cancer cells at various times throughout our lives, and that the immune system keeps them from developing into full-grown cancers. However, if a person eats a lot of sugar or takes drugs which lower the population of bacteria that normally keep the yeast population in check, Candida may grow beyond the immune system's ability to put it in place. It's an unfair burden.

BRYANT: So, although we usually think of bacteria as causing disease, in this case the bacteria are actually helping to maintain health by keeping a yeast imbalance in check.

McKEE: Yes. The bacterial population acts as a defense, but it can't survive the bombardment of antibiotics which we take in through pharmaceutical drugs or as residue in animal products.

We need to eat foods that are rich in bacteria, such as yogurt. And it's important to remember that if yeast isn't being fed lots of sugar, it doesn't have a nutrient source with which to grow rapidly. A low-sugar diet helps maintain a balance, so that the immune system doesn't have to work so hard.

BRYANT: I've come to associate Candida with women, primarily. Does it affect men as well?

McKEE: Yes, but Candida is fairly invisible, living primarily in the intestines. Women are often more aware of it because if they have the problem, they tend to get vaginal yeast infections. I suspect that those women have colonies in the bowel which, enjoying a lowered population of bacteria due to the antibiotics, move over to the vagina, where they show up clinically. That's just the tip of the iceberg, though. Many women who don't get vaginal yeast infections also appear to have the problem, and many men have the problem.

BRYANT: What kind of treatment is usually recommended for a chronic overgrowth of yeast?

McKEE: One of the difficulties we face is that Candida overgrowth is not recognized as a problem by many doctors. It's quite controversial. Physicians who actually recognize Candida as a problem usually prescribe a low-sugar diet to starve the yeast out, plus Nystatin—an antibiotic which kills yeast—or a stronger drug called Nizoral or Ketoconazole. Some doctors choose to use other substances with fungicidal activity. Someone involved in nutritionally oriented medicine would probably recommend a diet plan, plus an integrated program of supplements, which might include agents to strengthen the immune system; herbs like cloves and Pau D'arco and other substances that enhance the body's resistance to yeast; and bacteria like the acidophilus found in yogurt.

BRYANT: How is Candida usually diagnosed?

McKEE: There's no really reliable diagnostic procedure for it yet, but there are lots of methods that give us clues. For instance, you can do skin tests with a Candida antigen; you can do stool cultures. But often these methods simply don't work. The best test that I know of is a one-month trial of a comprehensive program designed to decrease the population of Candida. If you don't feel any different during that period of time, you don't have a problem with Candida. If you feel a lot better, or if you feel worse and then better, you probably do have a yeast overgrowth, and it would be very much worth investing six months working on it.

BRYANT: Has any literature been published on this subject?

McKEE: Yes. The two seminal works on the problem are *The Missing Diagnosis* by Orion Truss, M.D., which is very scholarly, and *The Yeast Connection* by William Crook, M.D. There's also a small pocket book by Shirley Lorenzani, Ph.D called *Candida Albicans, the Twentieth Century Disease*, put out by Keats Publishing. And the best cookbook resource that I've found for following the diet is *The Candida Albicans Yeast-Free Cookbook* by Pat Connally.

BRYANT: Is there another message you'd like to share about medicine, healing, and cancer in particular?

McKEE: We've made a great attitudinal mistake in viewing cancer as a vicious enemy to be battled with every weapon at our disposal. Just as infectious disease taught us to deal with our biological excrement, cancer can also be seen, and used, as a teacher trying to get a message through to us.

Cancer has taught and continues to teach us many of the secrets of life. In trying to find a cure for cancer, we've gained a greater understanding of genetic structure. And I think on a larger scale—socially—cancer has many messages for us, such as, "Let's make the biological, social and ecological health of the planet more of a priority than profit and power."

As individuals, cancer offers us a message about the way we spend our time. As life becomes more precious, we ask ourselves: Are we living in ways that reflect our values? Do we choose careers in order to impress others and gain approval, or do our careers exercise our healthy, creative impulses?

I think one of the many lessons cancer holds for us is that we need to find ways of detoxifying the poisonous byproducts of our industrial society rather than dumping them into the ocean or burying them in the ground and poisoning our environment with them. I'm certain that if we applied our scientific minds to it, we could find ways of converting highly toxic things into harmless, even useful substances. But it takes money, and it takes commitment of that money. Up until now we've favored the solutions offering short-term rewards. It may be cheapest to pay someone to dump toxic waste in a field somewhere in the middle of the night, but actions like this have created major ecological disasters.

I believe the greatest message cancer holds for us collectively is that we should face what the desire for higher and higher profits

is doing to our environment, our food chain, and our ways of being on this planet. I don't think we're going to make a lot of progress until we start listening to this message. I think we'll have cancer
until we learn the lessons cancer has to teach us.

BRYANT: What you're really calling for is a far-reaching educational campaign about disease and our relationship to the world.

McKEE: That's because I consider cancer to be a collective disease. It's not an individual disease.

One of the tenets of holistic healing is that we should all take
responsibility for our own health. That's good to a point, but I think
it's very wrong to tell a cancer patient that she's responsible because she didn't eat right or because she thought the wrong
thoughts or felt the wrong feelings, or whatever. We're all in it together.

The most successful cancer treatment programs I've been involved with have one thing in common. They all involve groups
of people coming together, supporting each other, and unifying
a belief system around whatever it is that they're doing. This works,
I think, because cancer comes from a very large collective energy,
and it will take large collective energies to deal with it.

Living and Dying with Unconditional Love

ELISABETH KÜBLER-ROSS, M.D.

Since the early 1960s, Dr. Elisabeth Kübler-Ross has worked with children and adults of all ages toward a greater understanding of death, dying, and transition phases of life. Recognized worldwide as a foremost authority in this field, she contributes to medical, social and spiritual efforts through individual and group counseling, workshops, her own scientific research, and writing for the general public. Since the international success of her first book, On Death and Dying, *which has been translated into over a dozen languages, she has written ten others, including* On Children and Death, Death: the Final Stage of Growth *and* AIDS: the Ultimate Challenge. *A founding member of the American Holistic Medical Association, and pioneer in the area of hospice care, Elisabeth Kübler-Ross travels extensively, offering lectures and five-day Life, Death and Transition workshops throughout the U.S. and in Europe.*

INTRODUCTION

In January, 1984, I attended a seminar on Death and Dying as part of a program offered by Maitreya Institute in Honolulu. I was impressed by the conference's focus on the process of dying, and with the panelists' willingness and ability not only to learn, but also to understand and communicate the concerns of the dying.

Elisabeth Kübler-Ross, who had participated anonymously, addressed the group at the seminar's closing. She talked about the importance of our work in trying to understand and let go of negativity, trying to live more fully, in touch with our emotions and our spirit. She finished with a warm "Keep up the good work."

Later, I introduced myself to Dr. Kübler-Ross and described my book in progress. She asked that we correspond and that I take her five-day workshop. In the months that followed, I arranged for a meeting with her at the new Elisabeth Kübler-Ross Center in Head Waters, Virginia.

Besides interviewing her on a professional level, I also asked several personal questions, based on how my parents and I had dealt with the pain and confusion experienced during my brother's illness with lymphoma and the process of his death. More than once during our exchange, she helped me to break through prejudices and limited viewpoints that I had not recognized in myself.

This allowed for a tremendous personal transformation to take place. I no longer felt the need to judge people who didn't want to "fight" their cancers. I no longer felt the need to prosyletize about my own preferred methods of treatment. Our meeting was a turning point for me, allowing me to approach future dialogues in a new and more gentle way, with an ear toward really listening, with no axe to grind.

DIALOGUE

BRYANT: As a health care practitioner and as an individual devoted to understanding and easing death as part of the life cycle, you work with many cancer patients. Your own personal experiences with cancer and other terminal disease must have helped to prepare you for the work you are doing today. Could you speak on your own first experience with cancer and how it has affected your development as a counselor?

KÜBLER-ROSS: It's hard to remember, really, what my first experiences with cancer were. My most impressive experience was with my brother-in-law. He had been married to my sister for only one year when he developed what they thought was an ulcer. I knew it wasn't an ulcer. I didn't know it intellectually, but intuitively I knew that it was cancer. So I told the doctor, who just got angry with me and said, "You're a typical medical student. This is your relative, so you imagine the worst." And I said, "I just absolutely *know* that this is more than an ulcer. He's not the ulcer type, and none of the ulcer diets or treatments help him." The doctor just laughed at me.

Well, finally I found an old-fashioned Swiss doctor with an open ear. He had given up his rural practice and had gone into surgery, but he was the kind of country doctor who really listened to people.

I went to him and asked him for a consultation. I said, "I'm in my last year of medical school, and I have intuitive knowledge that my brother-in-law has a very serious condition. Would you please give him a consultation?" So he saw my brother-in-law and immediately scheduled him for surgery. He allowed me to attend the operation, and when they opened him up, sure enough, he had a very rare cancer of the stomach lining which showed on the x-ray as if it were an ulcer. But by then it was so far spread that he only had a few months to live. That showed me that if I'd listened to my own intuition and if someone had heard what I'd tried to say, this man could have been saved. He died at age twenty-eight.

That was my first traumatic experience with cancer. We had no other cancer deaths in my family. After that, I went into medical practice and I saw many cancer patients.

BRYANT: How did this experience with your brother-in-law affect your future practice?

KÜBLER-ROSS: Well, I've emphasized listening to patients, trying to "hear between the lines." I believe that patients themselves know more than we doctors do. If they could only learn to listen more carefully to the intuitive knowledge coming from the spiritual part of their being, and listen a little less to the intellectual part, a lot more people could be helped. I'm sure of that.

BRYANT: How do we help people to listen to and follow their intuition?

KÜBLER-ROSS: That's been my life's work. During my five-day workshops I help people understand that human beings consist of physical, emotional, intellectual and spiritual aspects. We call these aspects of the self "quadrants," four parts of every human being, which we try to balance. The intellectual quadrant is most overdeveloped in our modern western society; the emotional quadrant is most damaged.

If we can repair the damage that is done to a human being before cancer begins to occur, if we can help a person to get rid of unfinished business — negativity and emotional traumas — then the spiritual quadrant opens up, and that person becomes very intuitive.

My own hope is that children might be raised in such a way that by the time they are teenagers, they are fully open to the development of their spiritual quadrant. My hope is that early on in life, they begin to know where they need to be, what their destinies are, what their life's work is. They shouldn't have to shop and shop around, searching till age thirty or forty without finding what they are supposed to know in order to fulfill their own destinies.

BRYANT: I've read about your technique of self-diagnosis. It seems to be a means of helping people to activate the dormant parts of themselves.

KÜBLER-ROSS: Yes. Jungian analyst Dr. Susan Bach has developed a very effective system of self-diagnosis based on a patient's own drawings. The drawings are evenly divided into four sections which correspond with the quadrants. We use the language of the spiritual quadrant in interpreting the drawings, because you have access to much more knowledge through the spiritual quadrant than you might ever get from your intellectual quadrant.

If you try to understand everything with your brain and you deny your own emotions, then your spiritual quadrant atrophies so that you can't hear your own inner voice, the voice of your own inner knowledge.

BRYANT: And with the knowledge that comes from inside, people are able to take positive steps in their lives.

KÜBLER-ROSS: Yes. Eighty-two percent of the people who participate in our five-day workshops experience positive, permanent life change. And the highest level of change consists of the participants' increased spiritual awareness.

For people who are in harmony with their own physical, emotional, intellectual and spiritual quadrants, death can be a graduation. Very simply, they die when they have learned their lessons — after they have taught and learned what they need to teach and learn. That's why some little children die. They've just come to be teachers of love and maybe some other quality. When they have taught what they wanted to teach, they are allowed to die. I no longer believe that death is an ending; I see death as a transition only.

BRYANT: Much of your work involves relating with people on a one-to-one basis, but through this educational process you've developed over the past twenty years, you've probably affected millions of people. Do you view your workshops as a means of changing society as a whole?

KÜBLER-ROSS: You can only change the world by changing yourself. I'm absolutely convinced of that. You can't change anything in the world if you don't start with yourself.

But if you learn to get rid of your total unfinished business, then you can become totally at peace — without any fear, without any anxiety, without any old hurts and traumas. And instead of criticizing others and condemning others and trying to change the whole world, the world actually does begin to change as your environment responds to you.

The people in your environment, including your children, your husband or wife, your boss, your friends and neighbors, all begin to see the development that takes place not only in you the person, but in your whole world. A person's love, compassion and understanding is a thousand times stronger than hate, anger and negativity. And it has incredible ripple effects as others around you learn to love as well.

Do you know Ken Keyes' story of "The Hundredth Monkey?"

BRYANT: I'd love to hear it again.

KÜBLER-ROSS: Not too long ago, it was observed that one hundred monkeys lived on a small island in the South Pacific. One day, apparently spontaneously, one of the monkeys washed her fruit before eating it. She repeated this procedure at the next meal, and perhaps because this practice eliminated some discomfort caused by sand in the fruit, other monkeys nearby began washing their

food as well. Soon, ninety-nine of the monkeys living on that island had acquired the food-washing habit. And at the very moment
that the hundreth monkey followed suit, a monkey of the same
species on an island more than seventy miles away began washing
his fruit.

The idea here is that if a certain critical number of people or
animals or any living creatures in the universe begin to change and
do a certain thing, then every single member of that species in
creation will begin to do that very same thing.

BRYANT: This story implies that we each have a role to play in
creating global conditions. Even something as utopian as world
peace becomes accessible as the result of personal practice.

KÜBLER-ROSS: Yes. And it works both ways. As long as we hate
and have wars in a great enough number, and as long as a great
enough number of people benefit from war and crime, we will have
an ever-mounting increase in war and crime. We have already seen
this in our universe. But if enough people stop thinking of war
and stop killing their fellow human beings and hating them, if a
critical number of human beings actually become loving, then li-
tle by little, all of the human beings on this earth will become loving and caring, compassionate and understanding. Then we will
have no problems with war—or with cancer either, for that matter.

BRYANT: Perhaps both the wars and the cancers we're experiencing today on such a massive scale are products of a value system
that needs to be examined closely.

KÜBLER-ROSS: We do so many destructive things, not only to
ourselves and to each other, but to mother nature—to this planet
Earth. And often we act destructively in the name of saving our
planet. For instance, take all the anti-war conferences and demon-
strations. The people involved ultimately want to save the earth,
but they are marching *against* something. They are *against* war.
They are *against* missiles. They are *against* nuclear weapons. *Against*
nuclear plants. Their motives may be very noble, but their being
against something instead of for something adds negativity. By
marching and shouting "no more war" they will never stop war.
They will only enhance the negativity which already surrounds us.

If you truly are doing something in the spirit of love, you do it
for the thing you love, not against something else. That is why,
to me, it seems as though the American Cancer Society unknowingly does a lot of harm as well as good. They go around and spread
fear. "Examine your breasts. Examine this and that. You are going

to get cancer if you're not careful." This is creating cancerphobia. People get frightened.

If someone were to do a very elaborate, detailed study of cancer statistics, I'm sure the incidence of cancer would be shown to increase in proportion to the prevalence of cancer prevention campaigns. The cancer rate goes up partly because people are filled with fear about cancer. And this fear of cancer actually contributes to the incidence of cancer.

BRYANT: And if we can get rid of the fear?

KÜBLER-ROSS: Then your chance of getting cancer or something like it is a thousand times decreased. When people really understand that even with cancer or some similar disease, they can live very lovingly and very creatively until they die, then the cancer rate will go down at a rate you wouldn't believe.

In the old days, people had the same phobia of TB. TB was rampant during the beginning of this century. Everyone was afraid. If someone had a cough, you suspected it was TB. Now it's cancer and AIDS. There will always be a disease which is especially frightening.

BRYANT: Have you ever envisioned a world without cancer?

KÜBLER-ROSS: I have often wondered what it would be like if there were no cancer. More people would become old and senile, sitting in nursing homes with strokes, unable to speak and unable to move—paralyzed.

Cancer does not have to be a nightmare. Cancer can even be turned into a blessing. It's what you make of what you have. That's the real issue.

BRYANT: Cancer as a blessing is a difficult image to come to grips with, but the concept seems an important one to investigate. Can you talk more about it?

KÜBLER-ROSS: Well, if I could choose a way to die, I would not choose to die quickly of a heart attack. I don't think that's ideal. It simply doesn't give your family time to adjust. You don't get to take care of the unfinished business. You don't have time to clean out your desk.

BRYANT: A lingering disease like cancer does give the patient time to reflect. And I have seen cancer help people to purge themselves of haunting negative attitudes and actions.

KÜBLER-ROSS: During the last twenty years, I've gotten hundreds of letters from people. For instance:

"The time since I got cancer has been the most blessed and richest time of my life, because suddenly I realized that all the things I worried about are unimportant. I worried about not being able to attend a country club function. I worried about my husband not being willing to buy me the right clothes. I would have been very upset a few years ago if we were not able to spend a winter in Florida. But now, these things seem totally irrelevant. Today, half an hour sitting with my husband at my side in the hospital room feeling totally content that we can look at each other and touch each other and communicate so fully with each other is worth more than a hundred vacations in Florida."

I get that kind of letter all of the time.

BRYANT: That letter records the process of someone who has transformed herself. And yet what about the intense physical discomfort surrounding cancer? If you're in pain, it's really hard to keep an objective perspective about the source of your suffering or the possibilities of transformation.

KÜBLER-ROSS: Pain has been a big issue for me during the past twenty years that I have been working with cancer patients. A big part of the work we're doing in the hospice movement has to do with keeping cancer patients free of pain. The idea is to enable cancer patients to live pain-free and consciously. We can do that now. We don't use injections; they make the patient feel overdependent on someone else. Also, shots make you dopey so that you can't think clearly; and when you can't think clearly you can't share love and openness the way you can when you're fully aware.

It's very important for people to educate themselves about alternatives, and to discard the myths associated with morphine and other pain-controlling drugs. If people are afraid of using morphine because of the social stigma associated with its abuse, dying people will suffer. If people believe that patients should feel pain every four hours or so before taking a pain-relieving drug, dying people suffer.

BRYANT: You've found a form of morphine which kills pain while allowing patients to retain waking consciousness?

KÜBLER-ROSS: Yes. We're having great success in using an oral pain syrup every four hours, before pain has a chance to recur. It's a very effective morphine elixir. Using this medication on a regular basis before pain sets in, the patient can then sit up comfortably or rock in a rocking chair during the last weeks of life. She's not dopey. She can have her dog at her feet and enjoy having her children and grandchildren around. She smells the breakfast smells at home—even if she can't swallow any more.

As soon as someone has intractable pain, that person can be put on the oral pain medication. We have people who have been on it for over a year. They don't get addicted, and they don't overdose with it. They have time to really function and live fully until they say goodbye. Hospices all over offer this kind of pain treatment today. It allows patients to fully experience their last months or weeks of life.

BRYANT: This pain treatment is used for people who are resigned to die within the next few months?

KÜBLER-ROSS: There is a big, big difference between resignation and acceptance. These people haven't resigned, haven't given up hope. They've simply accepted their situation honestly and openly.

BRYANT: Of course, you're most closely involved with the hospice movement and with people living the last stages of life. And understandably, a great deal of attention is being placed on comforting terminal patients in their final days. But I'm especially concerned with people who have, for instance, just discovered that they have cancer. It seems that if we could deal with patients' fear and pain at that point, then we could alleviate a great deal of suffering throughout the entire illness. For instance, most newly diagnosed cancer patients suffer terribly just facing the prospect of looking for medical care which will be responsive to their needs. So much is new. So much is unknown, unfamiliar territory.

KÜBLER-ROSS: Searching for the right physician can be very rough, just as it is hard to find an honest lawyer or a dentist that you love and trust. Very hard. If you are diagnosed as having a malignancy, you have to shop around for the best information. Who is the physician who listens? Which physician doesn't push a guilt trip on you when you don't want chemotherapy? You have to shop around. You ask people who have had cancer: friends, neighbors, family members. Who can help to create your support system? That's how you best find out.

BRYANT: One problem is that so many people feel obligated to take treatments like chemotherapy and radiation. So many people have a mistrust for anything that is not conventional, high-technology medical practice. Even people who have been exposed to other methods of treatment feel a certain sense of duty to provide their loved ones with the "best money can buy," which is usually the most expensive treatment—whether or not it's right for the patient. They seem to seek out security through what they perceive as "the established cancer treatments" such as surgery, radiation and chemotherapy.

KÜBLER-ROSS: Then maybe that's what they need to experience. Who are you to know what is good and what someone else needs to experience? We all have to choose and accept that which feels personally most comfortable for us. If someone needs to go through surgery, chemotherapy, everything, maybe that's the experience that's needed most at that particular time in that person's life. You must keep in mind that any treatment will help someone if the person being treated believes in it. Anything you believe in, anything you trust, will have positive, beneficial results.

I saw this at a drug clinic at Montefiore Hospital in New York, where we did lots of placebo studies. We used a great variety of drugs there in order to find out what is the best drug for which patient. And we treated them openly and honestly. If they trusted that we really meant well, if they believed that we were doing what was best for them, we got good results, no matter what drugs we used. The physical substances were almost irrelevant. On the other hand, if the patients did not believe in or trust what we were doing, we saw negative results.

We can observe this happening on so many levels. Let's say you smoke cigarettes. If you're afraid of your own smoking, and the people around you say, "Ooh, you're going to die of lung cancer," and make you irritable every time you light up a cigarette, then that preaching is doing much more harm than the cigarette would do if you were just relaxing with a cigarette, enjoying it.

The real question is, what helps you? What is good for you or bad for you? It's not so much the treatment you choose; it's your attitude about it.

BRYANT: So you don't discourage patients who believe one hundred percent in what the medical establishment has to offer, even if the treatment itself may be quite dangerous.

KÜBLER-ROSS: Of course not. And yet I also have patients who say things like, "A friend of mine has taken laetrile or acupuncture or vitamin C treatment, and he did terrific. How would you feel if I tried that?"

I simply say, "You do what's right for you. I'm not here to tell you what's good for you, because you know better than I do. I can tell you statistically how many have been helped by this approach or that approach. But you are not a statistic. You're an individual. So go for the method you trust, the method that feels right for you, with my blessings. And I will help you with support in whatever way I can. You and your own soul, your inner knowledge and feelings know."

Those patients do terrifically. Not all of them are helped physically, you understand. Not all of them get well. But maybe the purpose is not always to get well. Healing does not mean only to get well physically. Healing means to become whole before you die — to have the chance to learn all of your lessons.

BRYANT: By this definition, the healing process involves every aspect of a person's makeup.

KÜBLER-ROSS: Yes, and it's an unending process. In that process, it's important not to impose one's will on another. There are those who impose their will out of a sense of obligation. The families of cancer patients are often afraid that if the patient does not go "by the book," any worsening of their loved one's condition will be their fault.

Many cancer patients say, "I'm totally opposed to any more chemotherapy, but if I tell my doctor that, he'll drop me like a hot potato." That reflects the attitude of doctors who try to limit patients according to their own prejudices. But there are physicians who do not impose their will on their patients. They can hear the inner needs of their patients. They're flexible and open, and offer alternatives.

Bernie Siegel is a marvelous example of that. He came to my workshop, and at first he thought it was a little bit hocus-pocus — especially our idea that with spontaneous drawing we could tell what a patient's unfinished business is.

But, as I mentioned earlier, drawing whatever comes from your own intuition, when you're not thinking, gives you the cue as to where you're at and what one's unfinished business is. So we ask people to draw spontaneous pictures. We then read the pictures and suggest which issues each person should be working on. That was a little bit too far-fetched for Bernie Siegel, until I happened to read his picture.

Well, I didn't know anything about him previous to that encounter, but I was able to tell him what his unfinished business was — what he needed to work on. He was quite impressed.

Then he went home and repeated the exercise with his family. And each family member really started to work on his or her own unfinished business. One year later, Dr. Siegel came back to the workshop as a visitor with a slide presentation of what he'd done.

BRYANT: Would you say that most medical professionals could benefit a great deal from your workshops?

KÜBLER-ROSS: Yes. One recommendation we make to physicians is that, after finishing up their regular lab and diagnostic work, they also encourage patients to do some spontaneous drawing. This will show what emotional issues are adding to the patient's ill health.

Dr. Siegel did that for one whole year with all his cancer patients. He learned to accept them and their intuitive knowledge. Helping them resolve their unfinished business, as revealed by the drawings, was part of the healing process. His patients got better like you wouldn't believe! His work shows an understanding that getting cancer patients well means more than just improving physical health. It also involves helping people to live fully until they die.

BRYANT: The kind of life and the kind of death that you're describing for cancer patients seems to be available only to those people who fully accept their condition. What about the people who fight their cancers up to the end in hopes of "beating" the disease?

KÜBLER-ROSS: A person's dying with dignity does not necessarily mean dying nicely, quietly, in a state of acceptance. That's often a therapist's illusion. We want to be able to say, "My patient died peacefully. I must have done a good job." But that's just an ego trip for the health care professionals.

For a human being to live and to die with dignity means to die in character, and to be respected and accepted for that character. Now if all your life you've been a fighter, someone who always gets things done in your own way—which may or may not be the approved way of proceeding—then a dignified way of continuing to live with cancer, and of dying, would involve this same characteristic.

The goal for all of us is to love unconditionally. That is really the main ingredient of life. That's what we are in the physical world for: to learn and to practice unconditional love.

BRYANT: Constrained by the pressures of time and money, this must represent a tremendous challenge for the medical doctor.

KÜBLER-ROSS: Yes, but practicing unconditional love with your patients is really such a simple thing. If you have a fighter and a rebel, you just let him be a fighter and a rebel until he dies. That means, you don't go by his room saying, "There's that SOB in room

7B. He's going to give me a hard time again, so I'll skip him." Or if he starts complaining about some things that may actually need to be changed, you don't sedate him until he's too dopey to complain. You help him to externalize and express his anger. You may be surprised to see that this patient becomes the most adorable, loving patient of all.

BRYANT: What would you say is the most important thing for someone who works with the terminally ill to remember? What is the goal of the doctor who tends to the terminally ill?

KÜBLER-ROSS: Well, certainly your goal is not to prove your medical competence. Nor is it that every patient die quietly and peacefully. Your goal is that every patient be your teacher, teaching you to practice unconditional love. That means that you accept their personalities, no matter how obnoxious they seem to you. If you find that someone is obnoxious, it simply means that he or she pushes a button in you which has to do with your own unfinished business — either an obnoxious part of yourself or the reminder of an obnoxious, nagging relative, or whatever. But it's your own trip. It is very important that you understand that.

BRYANT: Some of the things you've said about unfinished business make me wonder if there is a particular character or personality that seems to attract cancer or other types of diseases.

KÜBLER-ROSS: I can't say that a certain personality is more likely to get cancer. I would say that someone who is terribly afraid of cancer is more likely to get it, because we usually end up confronting our biggest fears.

BRYANT: Before coming here, I sat down at two different times to prepare questions to ask you. My second set of questions had to do with the cancer and death of my eldest brother, Fred, who died in July of 1981. He was forty-eight years old.

KÜBLER-ROSS: My identical triplet sister was just diagnosed as having an inoperable brain tumor, so I'm in the midst of that now myself. And she's in terrific shape. When she was told that the expectation for her survival was one year at the most, and that if they operated she might have two years as a vegetable, her reaction was, "Let's go traveling. Let's see all the things I've always wanted to see."

BRYANT: Fred was following the Hippocrates Living Foods diet, which was very effective for him. But after months of following it successfully, he chose to share compassion with loved ones by accepting different kinds of foods: refined foods, cooked foods, meat—what we might consider the normal American diet. Gradually, he went off the Hippocrates diet, and eventually he abandoned it completely, even as his condition worsened. He died a very noble death, only thinking of others. I think he was very successful at purging himself of some of his unfinished business.

Several of the questions I've asked you today were inspired by Fred and the things we both went through, from the time that he first called me to say, "I have cancer. Don't tell anybody," right up to his death.

Reflecting on my brother's process, I remembered one verbal altercation he had with our father. All the stuff that had gone on between them for forty-eight years suddenly came out into the open. Fred did everything but hit him physically. A few days later, I tried to help them see how that blow-up had really been part of a cleansing process, and preparation for a new level of living. And slowly, over many months, wounds were healed. It turned out to be a very healthy situation.

Then, just two days before he died, after never having made any demands upon me during his illness, he called me up and demanded that I be in touch with another brother and get him to reconcile his differences with our parents. He requested that all of us seven brothers and sisters be in harmony. So I got on the phone to the others, and we all communicated that night—and then he died. He took care of some unfinished business and was able to use his process to help the entire family.

KÜBLER-ROSS: Now in this case, don't you think cancer came as a blessing? A sudden heart attack or accident would have left him with so much unfinished business.

BRYANT: Yes. I *have* experienced such blessings, not only through my experiences with my brother, but also with my grandfather, the Karmapa, and other loved ones with cancer.

KÜBLER-ROSS: We have to remember that in terms of illness, or in terms of life, it's not what happens to you that is important, but what you make of what happens to you—your attitude and your response. Everything that happens to you in life can be turned into a growth and learning experience. This is especially true with cancer.

Read my book, *To Live Until We Say Goodbye*. It shows how very much these people have learned and grown through their illnesses. You'll see how so many have become so creative, how they have become teachers of others through their own cancers. That's the potential of every illness, but we've been conditioned to associate cancer only with suffering, pain and horrors.

BRYANT: Rationally, I know that fear of cancer is partially our fear of death, and partially due to our own lack of understanding about the disease. But there must be more. Could you talk about the reasons for such widespread cancerphobia in today's society?

KÜBLER-ROSS: The reasons for our fears vary as much as human beings vary. If your grandfather with cancer died a dignified death at home, surrounded by his family, able to communicate and talk without his life turning into a nightmare, then fear of cancer may not be too great. It's another story if your experience with cancer came through someone who died after having gone shopping around from doctor to doctor, taking radiation treatment and one surgery after another, perhaps experiencing radiation burn. Or maybe the person you knew was not diagnosed until it was too late. Maybe then he tried chemotherapy and experienced the nausea and vomiting and hair loss without being prepared. If that's your past history, and then another person in the family gets cancer, all the ideas and experiences that came of your first cancer experience will be brought up again. You pass your own fear on to the patient, and the whole family becomes chaotic.

BRYANT: Unfortunately this oftentimes is the case. So it's extremely important that children be exposed to illness and death in a loving, open environment.

KÜBLER-ROSS: This is why I stress the importance of educating the children. If someone in the family has cancer, the young children should participate in caring and loving and whatever else is necessary to show them early on that cancer does not have to turn into a nightmare of isolation.

Of course there was a time when we didn't have adequate pain medication, and there was a time not too long ago, before I started my work, when cancer patients were not told the truth about their condition. People did not level with them. Their families whispered. They were isolated.

How would you like to be surrounded by people in a conspiracy of silence? Imagine knowing that you are dying, and that you are looking more and more horrible, while your family and best friends—people you have always loved and trusted— lie to you, saying, "You look great today. You're getting much better."

This has all changed tremendously during the last twenty years. Today, we have so many hospices available; we have even started

Children's Hospice International, so that we have all this available to youngsters. Things have changed one hundred percent. But there is still a tremendous amount of fear surrounding cancer. Everywhere, we learn that cancer is out to get us.

BRYANT: Several times during our conversation you've brought up the subject of hospice, which is for those people who are at the stage of dying...

KÜBLER-ROSS: The hospice not only benefits people who are dying, but also the family members—the husband who feels that he may not have the physical strength to take care of his wife or his father or another relative or friend. Hospice gives such people a break.

The hospice also supports the inner knowledge of patients—the knowledge that they have the right to call it quits when they no longer wish to prolong their lives with more surgery or more chemotherapy or more whatever. Hospice has been designed to offer unconditional love while taking care of patients' physical, emotional and spiritual needs.

More hospices crop up every year. More and more people are thankful that there is finally a place where others will accept them and not put guilt trips and pressures on them to take more and more treatment, when they themselves know that their days are numbered. That is a tremendous relief to a human being.

And think about the old woman whose husband has cancer. She can barely lift him; she can't stay up and take care of this person twenty-four hours a day. That's not humanly possible, no matter how much love there is in one's heart. So the hospice represents a tremendous relief. She knows that if her strength runs out, if she gets so worn out that she can no longer hear him, she can put him in a hospice for a week or two and recharge her own battery or wait until a grown-up son has a two-week vacation and can pitch in a little too. Places like this are a tremendous help. The hospice may take a lot of fear away from family members. And the dying patient needn't be afraid that he is such a burden that his wife will collapse of exhaustion before he dies himself.

BRYANT: A couple of times while you've been talking, even though I've been focusing on your words, I have experienced moments of great anger—feeling like a bomb ready to explode.

KÜBLER-ROSS: And what triggers that anger?

BRYANT: I've been having trouble with your idea of accepting one's condition and not fighting one's cancer full-steam ahead. At this point, I think my own conditioned resistance to what you've been saying is starting to break down. I'm on the verge of feeling receptive to your attitude of acceptance. I see that fighting what is real, like the demonstrators who choose to fight *against* war instead of *for* peace, will only add negativity to the world. But the process of confronting this change of attitude in myself makes me feel explosive inside.

KÜBLER-ROSS: The workshop group would be a greatly therapeutic process for you, just as your writing may help you sort things out and make sense of your brother's death.

Our workshops have involved people from an eleven-year-old child dying of cancer to a 104-year-old woman. And we've found over and over again that you can change any pattern in a couple of days, if the desire is strong. It doesn't have to take five years of therapy four times a week. You can change any negative pattern—any pattern which is not beneficial to your whole being.

BRYANT: I know someone whose attitude needs a change. I love him and want him to change for his own good. What can I do?

KÜBLER-ROSS: If someone doesn't want to change, that's fine. That's his or her choice. You can only be a catalyst. You can never impose your needs on someone else, no matter how close you are.

I mentioned earlier that a therapist's own need to look good professionally will often cause her or him to push for a "successful"—meaning peaceful—death. But that may not be the most dignified way for someone to die. The real test is to love others just the way they are, with all of their shortcomings. That is unconditional love.

You ask someone three times. Anything. Any question, any favor, you ask someone no more than three times. If you ask more than three times, you end up doing more harm than good by trying to impose your will upon someone. By pushing someone in this way, you're adding more negativity to yourself, since you become frustrated and angry. You're also making the recipient of your request angry, feeling pushed. Trying to change someone causes more negativity than you can imagine. If any human being has heard something three times from one person, that human being knows what is desired. That person must have the courage to say, "It's my life and my choice."

BRYANT: In other words, it's wrong to impose your will on someone else.

KÜBLER-ROSS: Right. The biggest negative trip you can place

on someone is to impose your will. Because in doing so, you're try-ing to deprive that person of the greatest gift human beings have been given by God—that is, free will. Free choice. If you nag or beg or demand, then you're being negative, no matter how posi-tive you think you are being. And that action will be evaluated very negatively after your own death. It's putting your own trip—your own needs—onto someone else, somebody with an entirely differ-ent destiny. You do not know what the real needs of another are; you do not know of the growth experiences needed by another.

It is always the patient who must make the decision. No one can choose for another. In the case of your brother, he was a grown-up man. He had to make his own decisions. You could offer him suggestions: where he might get some help, how he might prolong his life. But whether he accepted that was his own free choice. A gift of love is a gift without expectation.

BRYANT: What can I tell my mother and father? What can I say to help them accept what's happened in our family—the loss?

KÜBLER-ROSS: I don't know if there is anything you can say to them. You can only set an example. Maybe they have to learn to hurt. Maybe they have to learn to look at themselves. Maybe they have to look at all the things that they regret and that they haven't done. And through that pain they will grow.

We have a saying at the Elisabeth Kübler-Ross Center: "If you shielded the canyons from the windstorms that erode the rocks, you would never see the beauty of the carvings." Look at people who have gone through lots of trauma. They're the grand canyons—the most beautiful human beings in the whole world.

If your need is to protect people from going through their pain, then you're doing them a disservice. You're cheating them of their own growth experiences. All you can really do is love them. You can give them books to read. If they're ready to read them, they will. But they have to go through their own school. You can't go to school for them, any more than you could go to school for a child. Children have to go for themselves, every day. That way they learn and grow. They become stronger and able to cope with things. Taking that experience away from a child is not love. Love is know-ing when to put the training wheels on a child's bicycle, and then also knowing when to take them off. *That* is what love is all about.

Seventeen Days Before Farewell

JULIAN BECK

Actor, director, philosopher and writer, Julian Beck was a master of communication. Having begun his career as an abstract painter, he decided to dedicate himself to revolutionary theatre. He began by designing innovative sets, which influenced the use of theatrical space throughout the Western world.

In the 1950s, Julian Beck and his wife Judith Malina created the Living Theatre. From the beginning of the Off-Broadway movement in New York and throughout the decade, they packed small theatres with poets, artists, filmmakers, dancers and musicians. Reflecting Julian's and Judith's commitment to collective process, the Living Theatre presented collectively written works for twenty years, challenging their audiences by breaking with social and aesthetic conventions. Best known works of the Living Theatre's repertoire include The Brig, Paradise Now, Prometheus at the Winter Palace, and The Archeology of Sleep, which were performed in Europe as well as in North and South America.

Beck's poems, plays and other works have been published in several languages. As an actor in his last years, he enjoyed critical acclaim in roles for movies and television.

INTRODUCTION

Although I had not met Julian Beck before our interview, we shared many friends and experiences, and I had a great sense of trust, respect and appreciation for his life's work. In fact my own work as an environmental artist drew great inspiration from the Living Theatre. Through a mutual friend who considered Julian to be his mentor, I learned of the inner workings and depths of this innovative system of communication arts. This served as a foundation for my exchange with Julian. And from the beginning of our meeting I sensed a deep, mutual understanding, and the familiar warmth of friendship.

I arrived at the home of Julian Beck and Judith Malina on a hot, humid day. Entering their old, oversized apartment filled with theatre posters, Julian's paintings, props, manuscripts, and human activity was like stepping into a Living Theatre production. Every particle of space, dust and motion seemed to be a meaningful part of the total statement.

From the outset, I was aware that I was sitting in the presence of a great artist and human being who was fighting for his life. Although he was experiencing great suffering throughout our exchange, when I asked him if he wanted to stop, he insisted upon continuing. Not only did he push himself to go beyond the pain in order to respond to my questions, he was also extremely aware of and responsive to the needs of the audio-video technicians. And he communicated his experience with the skill and passion of a great actor.

Throughout our exchange, I sensed the bliss as well as the anguish of a unique human being, a performer who gave of himself not only as a means of self-expression, but also as a means of benefiting others.

The following day, Julian Beck had his last chemotherapy treatment. He died sixteen days later on September 14, 1985.

DIALOGUE

BRYANT: How has being confronted with the prospect of death by cancer affected your life? Your notion of sanity? Your notion of death?

BECK: When I was first confronted with the fact that I might die of cancer, I immediately thought of the fact that we had no money in the bank, the fact that I had a lot of unfinished writing, and that the Living Theatre didn't have a base any more. Plus, certain things had to be said about burial: where and how. So I began to attend to as many of these things as I could.

I was really lucky, because a lot of film and television offers came to me at that time. I worked a great deal on *The Cotton Club, Poltergeist II,* and *Miami Vice* because I wanted there to be some money in the bank to take care of the family's needs, just in case the angel of death should descend at some moment, unforeseen.

Also, I've been trying to work on my own writing. I've readied two plays for publication, and I'm working on my book *Theandric,* while writing poems, getting my thoughts out, trying to attend to my daughter's education, and my granddaughter's. I must be prepared to face this eventuality, yet just as the Zen Buddhist monk laughs at the moon, I have to find a way of laughing at death.

BRYANT: It appears that you're using this experience to take care of a lot of loose ends. You certainly seem to have understood the monk's laughter.

BECK: You know, three days after I was hospitalized, Allen Ginsberg came in and said, "How does it feel to be dying?" And I said, "Who's dying? I happen to be ill, but I have no intention of dying. I have much too much to live for, too much to do and experience and experiment with. I'm madly in love with life right now." And at that time I was really very sick. He said things to me like, "After all, in sixteen million years we're going to disappear into another black hole. The sun is going to explode and become a supernova."

BRYANT: It's important to always remember impermanence but we're here today, dealing with the here and now.

BECK: Right. That's my feeling. We're here today, right now. What happens in sixteen million years is of great interest, but it really has no practical application to my condition tonight. I want to concentrate fully on my life — my loves, my work, my art.

The doctor says to me that with my attitude and my physical

progress, I make his work worthwhile. And that's encouraging. But I have to say each day, "Today may it be true, may I truly be progressing. Let us hope." There are all these favorable signs, but one just doesn't know. One lives in a world of uncertainty. Some call the uncertainty the cancer concentration camp—the "ccc"—because indeed, you're living with the knowledge that there is a sword hanging over your head all the time.

Nevertheless, you have to live. If you stagnate, surely you give death free reign. And the longer you feel involved in the world, the stronger is the confrontation and the possibility of attaining success in this struggle.

I am wrestling with the angel of death twenty-four hours a day, and still, I smile and bow low, and say, "I am not yet ready for you."

BRYANT: As an innovative actor/director involved with raising consciousness of social issues, and as an artist devoted to poetry and theatre, can you talk about how your experience with cancer has acted as a tool to help you strive toward "truth" in your discipline?

BECK: We need to come together to celebrate life, not to invoke death. When Freud spoke of the death wish, he spoke psychologically, but I think this wish today is rooted in the unpleasantness of our social system. People would just as soon die as try to live.

During my illness, I've been surrounded by a very valuable, loving support system. And I've become more aware that we should be treating each other this way all the time, all our lives, in all of our activities, with this much delicacy, this much caring, and this much discipline. *We have to establish loving support systems with each other.* I would like to make this clearer through the theatrical work, in the art that we produce, and through all of our creations.

So it's for everyone to work on. We have to find, through every means of creative expression, ways of making this statement with power—forcefully. We've got to be able to break through the walls that prevent us from seeing.

BRYANT: The walls—you mean our conditioning?

BECK: Yes. We don't want to die, but we also don't yet believe that we have to support each other's lives, protect each other, care for each other, or help provide ourselves with a healthy atmosphere. We're poisoning the entire planet. We're crazy. We're invoking death.

BRYANT: Why?

BECK: I think because life is for most people so difficult, so burdensome, so devoid of meaning, so painful, that people have come to hate life and would just as soon destroy it as not—would just as soon go to war and be killed as not. And this has got to change, because it can only lead to the death of our planet.

The water is going to go soon; the air is going to go. The ecologists have warned us. Each day, our food supply system pours into the body a load of artificial chemicals, preservatives and other elements which only stress the body. Instead of nourishing us, they eat away at the core of our being. It's part of the death invocation.

We can't continue to manifest ourselves as a people who love death more than we love life. Working in theatre, we can strive to evoke a sense of hope, a sense of love, a sense of community—mutual support. Because if we can support each other, we can also support ourselves.

BRYANT: Is this the sort of thing you're writing about now?

BECK: Yes. I mentioned my book, *Theandric*. The title is an old English word signifying the presence of the divine (Theos) and man (Andros). I feel that today the soul and the spirit have been driven into obscurity. It makes me think of the *oubliette*, a kind of underground jail, covered with a grill so that the prisoner was essentially forgotten. There was no longer any kind of communication with the prisoner except the daily bread and water. And I feel that we've done this to our souls, and that's why we can't perceive, we can't judge, and we can't feel anymore. We've become a feelingless people, and we have to restore feeling if we're going to create a network of life support. I see art and culture as playing a very important role here.

BRYANT: Can you talk more about how your illness has affected your family and others close to you, and how they have affected you?

BECK: I've always been a lover. I love people. I love to embrace and to touch and to hug. I love the sensuality. After I found out I had cancer, I felt tremendously inhibited suddenly. But now I'm able to express more in the house, in the family and with friends. I sense a much greater openness than ever before. Many people don't realize how important family and other means of support actually are to the person who is ill. I really hope that the importance of home-based support can be proven in a scientific way.

BRYANT: Can you talk about how you and your loved ones reacted when you first found you had cancer?

BECK: I remember I was with Judith. We were married thirty-five years at the time. I'm sure I turned pale in the doctor's office.

We got into the car and just sat and talked for half an hour. Judith said right away, "You've got to fight this." And I said, "I'm going to." We talked about ways to do it.

We had been commissioned by the French government to do a new play, which we were to take on tour. So I worked on writing, putting together the collective ideas of the group, creating *The Archeology of Sleep*. I battered away at the typewriter and finished the play at about one o'clock in the afternoon one day. We all drove into Nantes, and went to the theatre. I read the play to the company, and there was great enthusiasm. Then I picked up my bag and went to the hospital for my operation. So the company went to work on the play by themselves, with Judith there to direct.

A curious thing happened then. And I should preface this by saying that neither Judith nor I have ever been sick a day in our lives. Well, Judith was having a pain in her side and had gone to male doctor after male doctor, all of whom told her, "It's just a neurosis. It's not anything real." Well, finally we found a doctor in Nantes who said, "Oh my God, you have to be operated on immediately. Your gallbladder is about to burst. So she went into the hospital too. We had adjoining rooms, and she was there for almost two weeks. They removed her gallbladder and gave her a gallstone as a trophy."

Meanwhile, the company rallied marvelously. They would come to the hospital for advice and to go over staging with Judith and the scenic appurtenances with me. It was a kind of heroic period. We got out of the hospital with about five or six days to go before the opening, and the opening was marvelous. The play was beautiful and extremely well liked.

BRYANT: So from the beginning you were surrounded by a loving, supportive community of family and friends.

BECK: Absolutely. If left alone by my family, if forsaken, that would have been a terrible blow. If I'd felt that my family had given me up for dead, I would've been wiped out, as if the props had been taken out from under me.

Here in New York, I have the great fortune of being surrounded by people I love. There's Judith, and two children who are grown up now but very close. My daughter comes to me when she's not in school to hug and embrace me — to ask if there's anything I want, if there's anything she can do — and we sit and have conversations more than we ever have before about her life, her career, her schoolwork, her loves....

During my last stay in the hospital, Judith called all our friends and said, "Come to the hospital." It was like a party in that hospital room. There were people there all the time, and the whole wall got covered with greetings and drawings. People gave head massages and foot massages almost every day, which seemed to evoke all of the restful, sleepy elements of the body. It was wonderful. My time there passed with a sense of being much loved. One friend came and said, holding my hand very tight, "We're not going to let you go." That's how it felt.

And the support system has grown. Hanon Reznikov and Ilion Troya of the Living Theatre live with us in the apartment, and they've both been marvelous in relieving me of quotidian duties and making things very light, gay, attractive, and easy. When I'm feeling lonely, rejected and neglected, my support system is like a hundred strings attached to me, pulling me up to the light.

BRYANT: How have you experienced the fear? How has the fear of death affected the people in your life?

BECK: Initially they were all very frightened. But then my wife said, "If anyone could beat cancer, it ought to be you." And Judith has been just terrific. She was at the hospital every day, from morning till they threw her out at ten or eleven at night—always encouraging me to get strong, take it easy, saying, "Don't worry about work or anything. I'll take care of it."

This has been enormously helpful. That's why I say I'm very fortunate. I think the cancer, and the fear, brought us all closer together. We began to be conscious of the need to create a network—a life support system, planet-wise. It's one of our great social and political needs.

BRYANT: Since you have been a cancer patient, how would you describe your own role in your healing process?

BECK: When I first found that it was cancer, in March of 1983, I asked how long the cancer had been growing. The doctor thought anywhere from two to three years. I immediately calculated that three years earlier, there had been three very significant events in my life. The most significant was the loss of the person I was in love with, who said one day, "It's over. I'm going away." Then, just one week later, my mother died. We had had a very good, solid relationship. Then when I returned to Europe, I began working like crazy on The Yellow Methuselah. It was five months of the most strenuous work imaginable: building and painting the set, making the hundred and fifty costumes. I hardly slept at all. I didn't eat. My body was under tremendous stress.

Finding out I had cancer, I made the connection between that stress and my health. I realized immediately that I had to change my form of life. I had abused myself, and felt abused by the world, so I simply had to take greater care of myself. And that has been part of the therapy.

BRYANT: Once you realized that your lifestyle and behavior patterns contributed to your condition, what were some of the changes you made?

BECK: I used to disregard the messages of my body. It was as if I were a car that was going to run forever. I just wanted to put my foot on the gas and go. Now I'm trying to cultivate my body and make love to it instead of treating it as a convenient machine. I'm trying to purify it and get rid of those elements of stress which have entered it in the past couple of years.

I'm meditating a lot. I go to the park, lie under the green trees, and bask a little in the sun. When I get tired I sit down, stretch out. I either close my eyes and meditate or I read, or I just float. Sometimes I meditate until I get into a white space where I'm just drifting, and this cools out my whole body. I remind myself twenty times a day to breathe.

And there are a dozen ways in which I try to give my body a new kind of care. Ilion is an expert Reichian masseur. At least every other night, he gives me a thorough massage. He locates the centers of tension, and he helps it all flow out of my body so that the immune system can do its work well.

Then there's the work I want to do. If I can do two to three hours of work each day—if I get a chance to work on my writing, on my other projects and correspondence—I'm very lucky. That's therapy too.

BRYANT: Apparently, you're involved with going beyond the physical aspects of your illness—working with lifestyle changes, the psychological elements, the setting of limits for yourself.

BECK: Oh yes. I have found out that the human body is a very delicate mechanism, and that we have to care for it. It needs a certain calm, a certain ease, and the right fuel.

You know, for twelve years I had eaten very little sugar. I had also stopped smoking for fourteen years. Plus, being a vegetarian for thirty-five years, and living with the Living Theatre tribe, whom I loved very much, doing the work that I loved, I was certain that I was impervious to such a thing as cancer. When the doctor said to me, "Absolutely it's cancer," I was stunned. I guess that's true for everyone. You think it will happen to someone else, but not you.

One of the doctors I spoke with said that the cures for cancer seem to work with people who try everything. For those people who resign themselves only to radiation, for instance, the therapy is less effective. That struck me as significant.

BRYANT: Can you describe one of the relaxation techniques you use?

BECK: When I started chemotherapy, I would get up every morning and go to a chair facing Central Park to do what I called my green meditation for about an hour. I also learned a Simonton-inspired meditation, visualizing my cancer being consumed by white blood cells. I feel this was very effective, and I still do it every day—in the morning when I awake, in the afternoon, and more or less before I go to sleep. As I'm lying there falling asleep, I visualize the healing process.

BRYANT: Physically, how do you feel or sense your immune system?

BECK: In the visualization meditations that I do, I try to direct the immune system. I try to locate the glandular secretions and the white corpuscles to see whether they're passive or active. I try to send them to the cancer cells. I feel that my immune system needs my strength, my relaxation and my meditation in order to function properly.

BRYANT: In what other ways did you take part in the process of your diagnosis and healing?

BECK: After the tumor was removed from my stomach, I felt that something was still there, growing. So the doctor did a sonogram and a CT-scan and x-rays, and everything—pancreas, stomach, liver, gallbladder, spleen—tested fine. But my stomach continued to swell up, and suddenly I couldn't eat anything. I vomited everything. Finally, the doctors admitted that something was wrong. I had a tumor that had attached itself to the omentum, the blanket of tissue that covers and supports the entire abdominal system. The cancer had moved there, and it was very serious.

So even as a patient, I'd had to analyze my illness. I told the doctors initially that something was terribly wrong, and then I told them that I wanted to know absolutely everything they knew. In fact, I think that if I hadn't pushed the doctor so much to find out what was going on, I might not have survived another two weeks.

BRYANT: Your illness has brought you through a process of transformation. You've been using your intuition and instincts to help
you understand the needs of your system. Can you talk about how
cancer has acted as a teacher?

BECK: Cancer is a stern teacher. It says essentially, "Do everything you can to get well. You are ill now. You are challenged; I
challenge you to throw me out the door." I don't know precisely
how people can be alerted to this, but I think greater exposure
should be given to the cancer patients who live beyond the famous
five-year "survival" limit. More and more, that limit is being sur-
passed, with people surviving ten, twelve, twenty-five years beyond
the time the cancer was first diagnosed. I think this has a lot to
do with the percentage of people who are trying many different
approaches to therapy and who are not giving up. I think the important thing is not to give up.

BRYANT: Can you talk about how cancer has been your teacher on a more personal level?

BECK: In a way, the cancer has taught me how to live. The process I've been following has been very gratifying, even fun. I had
been living in a way that was self-destructive, and I've found a gen-
tler way.
    Certainly it has awakened an awareness, to a greater extent than
I had before, of the imminence of death. We are all going to die.
It has helped to widen my consciousness about the sacredness of
the body and the need to attend to it. It's sad that I got to work
on these things only when the angel of death stood directly in front
of me.

BRYANT: Can you describe how personally being confronted with
cancer has acted as a means for you to review and reevaluate your
life?

BECK: I think that when you feel yourself being drawn into the
sphere of death, you begin to take account of what you've done,
how you've done it—and the changes affecting your personality.
Before I was aware of having cancer, I was given to shouting and
fits of anger. But I haven't raised my voice in two-and-a-half years.
That's how long it's been since I've felt on the outs with anybody.
If someone does something foolish, that's the way it is, and one
can deal with it. There is no reason to stir up inner anguish about
these things; we can simply alter our personalities. That, I've found,
is the easiest thing to do.
    When the doctor told me I had cancer, the change happened

to me as easily and as quickly as turning on a light switch.

BRYANT: Can you talk more about how the process of confronting cancer and reflecting upon your past has served as a means of letting go of unwholesome thoughts and deeds?

BECK: I think the cancer has made me aware of the things that poison me. It has pushed me toward a process of self-purification. Just as I turned on that light switch and got rid of the anger that had been part of my personality for so long, so I began to deal with all of life. Suddenly it was a great thing to be able to greet people on the street, thinking, "I'm so glad you're there." Suddenly it fills me with joy just to see sunlight.

BRYANT: So your experience with cancer has made you generally more aware.

BECK: The cancer has forced me to focus my attention on what I think of as the life-giving forces, rather than grinding away splenetically at all the things that are wrong. I still rail against them a lot, but mostly I do that in my writing, when I'm trying to make clear what kind of world we live in and how it has shaped theatre. I think this has been one of the favorable aspects of the cancer.

BRYANT: Elisabeth Kübler-Ross has said that cancer could be considered a blessing. Do you feel that the experience of dealing with cancer has been a healing or purifying process—a positive condition?

BECK: If it weren't such a killer, it might be easier to see the good side. But I guess the fact that it is a threat makes it a potential helpmate. Whereas we might otherwise live our lives wastefully, cancer teaches us to treasure and use every minute advantageously. We become more productive. When you find out that you're afflicted, you have the impetus and the ability to change the form and the ways in which you move, talk and relate to people. And I think that's a healer.

BRYANT: You appear to have made peace with many aspects of yourself during this period.

BECK: Yes, with myself, my loved ones and my home. But I have not yet made my peace with the military, or the state, or private property, or money—the economy—those things, no. And it's my pleasure to strive against these things and try to change them. That's my work.

BRYANT: We've talked about cancer, art, culture, and ways of looking at the world. The connection between our own health and the health of our society is too strong to ignore. It's tempting to equate the disease, cancer, with imbalanced states of being. As a member of our human family, as a communicator, and as a concerned person, how do you respond to the idea of cancer as a metaphor for what has gone wrong in our culture?

BECK: I think our culture is being eaten up alive by poisons, which are the side effects and the direct effects of our actions. The cancer of society is the result of our alienation from each other, our social and political enmity, our competitiveness, our sense of frustration — of not being satisfied, of not being able to get ahead in the world, and the struggle of it all. Society has innumerable tumors everywhere, which will kill us if we as a planet of people don't begin to heal our home, the earth. This must be made clear. It's the most important thing.

But people are so immune to reality, so alienated from it, that they neither believe nor care. Our work is to get through and to say, "Look, our world is dying of cancer. Now *what are we going to do?*" And we must go through those changes of healing and self-healing, to create a life-support system that will really work.

People have the habit of saying, "That's utopianism. It will never work." On this side of the world, they say, "The communists are bad. If we don't have the weapons, they'll come here and make us all into communist drones." Why can't we just say, "Look, we have two alternative systems, and a lot of stages in between." We need to find out which one is the most effective for each society, which system or combined system will best provide for our needs, which one is going to take care of our creative capacities, and which is going to provide us with the most loving environment for us to grow in. Some people will work to see whether or not capitalism is the most efficient way of producing gross wealth; others will work to see whether socialism is capable of producing enough space and room for happiness, individuality, and economic growth. And if neither system works, let's try something else.

The important thing is to try to find the answers artfully and in a kindly manner, for everyone's ultimate benefit — gently, in a soft way; not in the way of some macho patriarchy. We need to soften up — soften the tumor and make it shrink. We need to get to work on the purification of our daily lives. In this way, cancer is an appropriate metaphor for our condition.

Appendix A

RANGJUNG RIGPE DORJE
THE XVI GYALWA KARMAPA

The Gyalwa Karmapa, along with the Dalai Lama, is among those who share responsibility for the leadership and spiritual guidance of Tibetan Buddhist culture. After the occupation of Buddhist Tibet by China in 1959, the XVI Karmapa, the XIV Dalai Lama, and over one hundred-twenty thousand other monks and lay Tibetans went into exile as a means of ensuring their survival and preserving their culture. Arriving in India, the Karmapa—like the other great lamas—continued his work, teaching Tibetan Buddhist doctrine and the science of meditation.

Acknowledged as one who possesses the qualities of the Buddha of compassion, each Karmapa is a great scholar and meditation master. As the supreme holder of the Karma Kagyu* lineage of Tibetan Buddhism, he is believed to embody, represent, and guide its accumulated spiritual energy. The unbroken Kagyu lineage has been passed from teacher to disciple since the eleventh century. Received by heads of State throughout the world, the XVI Karmapa was one of the many lamas responsible for bringing Tibetan Buddhist philosophy and science to the West.

My association with Karmapa began in 1974. I had recently returned to Europe after having studied meditation and Tibetan Buddhist philosophy in Dharamsala India, and the Karmapa ordained me as a Buddhist monk. During the next few years, I studied under him and had the opportunity to travel as part of his

---

* The Kagyu lineage, like each of the four lineages of Tibetan Buddhism, is a vehicle for transmission of certain meditative teachings, particularly that of Mahamudra. Mahamudra guides the practitioner toward a realization of the true, awakened nature of mind, and helps the practitioner to transform all experience into understanding and skillful means.

entourage in Europe and the U.S. Feeling that I could be of more service to the American Buddhist community as a lay-person, I returned my monk's vows in 1977 but have continued to support Buddhist inspired projects in the U.S.

In 1981, I heard that the Karmapa was seriously ill with recurring stomach cancer, and that he was on his way to Hong Kong for treatment. Soon, he was transferred to the American International Hospital in Zion, Illinois, where he received the benefit of state-of-the-art medical technology and complementary medical practices. In spite of several serious health crises including kidney failure, disseminated intravascular coagulation, and pneumonia, he refused pain medication which might interfere with his ability to think and speak. On November 4, 1981, he was declared clinically dead, although he remained in the hospital for three days in a "post mortem" state of meditation before his physical body became cold.

At this time, I met with T'ai Situpa, also an eminent meditation master, and leader and lineage holder of the Kagyu tradition. During our talk, T'ai Situpa made the statement that the Karmapa's death would serve somehow toward bringing about a cure for cancer.

Having begun to investigate cancer as a means of learning about my brother Fred's illness, I was driven both by a need to understand the meaning of T'ai Situpa's words and by a desire to contribute to the process of "bringing about a cure."

At the time of our discussion, I assumed that he was alluding to technological breakthroughs in medicine. But as my investigation progressed, I became convinced that the real breakthrough leading to an understanding of and cure for cancer would come about through dialogue.

In fact, the Karmapa was the pivotal connection between myself and over half of the contributors to this dialogue-based work. It was at the Karmapa's cremation ceremony—at Rumtek Monastery in Sikkim, India—that I met with and interviewed West German physician Christian Kellersmann. And it was Dr. Kellersmann who referred me to Dr. Dwight McKee, who had served as the Karmapa's physician in the U.S. Dr. McKee introduced me to Dr. Emanuel Revici, with whom he was studying. Eventually Dr. McKee also presented me with the opportunities to contact and meet with Drs. Michael Lerner and Jacob Zighelboim.

I met with T'ai Situpa frequently as I investigated the reality of cancer both from scientific and psychological viewpoints. After one such meeting, at a conference on death and dying where T'ai

Situpa was the principal speaker, I met Dr. Elisabeth Kübler-Ross, who introduced me to the work of Dr. Bernard Siegel who, in turn, introduced me to Sigo Press.

And it was through the Karmapa's own illness that I came in contact with the Hippocrates program of healing with living foods, which led me to interview Dr. Ann Wigmore.

Surely it is no accident that this man who, after living all of his life in Tibet and India and then coming to the U.S. to teach, to undergo medical treatment and finally, to shed his physical body, should act as a bridge between Eastern and Western cultures. And it seems fitting that the Karmapa, a master of consciousness himself, would contribute as he has to our understanding of consciousness in relation to cancer.

For me, and for thousands of others, the Karmapa's life represented more than the life of one man. He was and is a symbol of great wisdom, compassion, and refined scholarship, qualities which reflect the heart of the Tibetan Buddhist tradition.

Appendix B

THE SCIENCE OF TIBETAN MEDICINE

A Personal Introduction to Tibetan Medicine

I've had many opportunities to learn about medicine first hand. As a teenager in the 1950s, I suffered from asthma. Experimenting with a restricted diet, I remember being astounded at its positive effect on my breathing and behavior. Then watching my youngest brother come close to death and go through tests, treatments, and four radical surgeries for Crohn's disease, I observed some of the best and worst aspects of Western allopathic medicine. I also witnessed my mother's ability to help heal my brother with relentless, caring devotion and determination. Watching my grandparents die, I gained insight into the meaning of loss, attachment, denial, deep suffering and pain, and I began to recognize my own lack of preparation for dealing with death.

My own cultural background simply didn't offer answers to my questions about sickness, dying and death. Those subjects were simply "not to be discussed" with family members and friends. This attitude encouraged fear in every instance of illness. I wanted more openness and communication on these issues, so in the early 1960s I began to search for answers beyond my own culture.

My interest in Tibetan medicine was sparked in 1974 while I was living as a student and practicing Tibetan Buddhist meditation in Dharamsala, India, where one sees the snowy Himalayan peaks. On the day of my arrival, I discovered that my passport and return airplane ticket had been stolen. The theft was news, and word spread fast. I was soon approached by a Westerner who told me of a Tibetan woman who had the mental power of determining the thief. Enthused, I followed his directions until I found her.

She turned out to be Dr. Lobsang Drolma, the famous Tibetan physician and director of the Tibetan Medical Institute. I told her my story as we walked up the mountain together, and Dr. Drolma did disclose the identity of the thief.

In the months that followed, various personal health problems found me lined up early in the morning with the Tibetan mothers, children, and Western travellers waiting to be diagnosed and treated by this doctor, who was said to possess the qualities of Tara, feminine aspect of the Buddha. The soft touch of Dr. Drolma's hands as she read my pulse, her radiant smile and patient concern always brought an instant sense of comfort. Completely dedicated to the art and science of healing, Dr. Drolma made house calls to see me and numerous other patients whenever illness prohibited travel. One day, while Dr. Drolma was off on a far-away, emergency house call, I sought consultation with Dr. Yeshi Donden, personal physician of the XIV Dalai Lama. In the months that followed, both Doctor Drolma and Dr. Yeshi Donden showed true compassion and concern for both my mind and my body; and the treatments they recommended were quite effective.

Coupled with the mind training of Tibetan Buddhist meditation, Tibetan medicine helped me to accept and develop a greater sense of responsibility for my own health. The Tibetan approach to medicine also helped me to perceive myself always in relation to my environment.

When I began work on this book, I felt a need to share the benefits of my own experience. While investigating various medical disciplines, I came to understand how information about the Tibetan system might contribute to a broadening of Westerners' perspectives on the form and function of medicine. Because Tibetan medicine is largely based on Ayurvedic and Chinese medical systems (the two major systems of the Orient), it seemed an appropriate place of departure for initiating and deepening cross-cultural medical dialogue.

Studying Tibetan medical texts in English, it becomes apparent that major discrepancies between Tibetan and Western medicine are based on differing systems of anatomical classification. Another major difference lies in the Tibetans' emphasis on the psychospiritual elements of medicine.

During the mid '80s, I met with and interviewed several Tibetan medical doctors, sometimes in the presence of Western physicians. It was exciting to listen to members of each group describe certain conditions from two entirely different perspectives. Often such discussions resulted in surprise and joy—the fruit of peeling back layers of language and culture in order to reach one shared conclusion.

Because the Tibetan system of medicine is practiced today much as it was over a thousand years ago, its integrity has been preserved. On the other hand, the fact that it is rooted in a culture so foreign to our own makes it hard for modern Westerners to understand, much less trust, understand and accept. The study of Tibetan scientific writings was a slow process which taught me a great deal about some of the underlying assumptions of both cultures.

The following is designed to reach scientifically oriented as well as lay readers from diverse cultural backgrounds. May it serve as a springboard for medical exchange on the levels of theory and practice.

Background

Tibetan medicine is a comprehensive system of health care based on a synthesis of the ancient Indian tradition of Ayurveda, the ancient Chinese system of astrology[1], the highly advanced Persian/Greek medical system, and indigenous shamanic Tibetan healing practices. Gyu-zhi, the basic, eight-volume Tibetan medical text, was written during the "golden age of Tibetan medicine," eighth to eleventh centuries A.D. Facilitation and maintenance of physical, intellectual and spiritual equilibrium is the primary goal of Tibetan medical practitioners.

Traditionally, the training of a Tibetan physician is a long and rigorous process, involving up to fourteen years of preliminary study, up to six years of medical school, and additional years of work as an intern, supervised by an experienced doctor. Although hundreds of pages of ancient medical texts, commentaries, and pharmacological catalogues must be memorized by every medical student, human qualities including skillful use of the senses, intuition, wisdom and compassion are considered to be as important as one's capacity to gather and memorize great quantities of information. Ultimately, compassion is considered to be the foundation upon which all medical practice rests.

The Tibetan doctor, thoroughly trained in pharmacology, is familiar with the ingredients in every medicinal formula he or she may prescribe. The process of choosing a medicinal formula involves identifying an individual's condition, and then identifying both the strength of the individual and the strength of the person's disease. After comparing these variables, the physician will try to create a medicinal compound to "match" both the person and the disease. The physician's ability to choose the proper medicine requires knowing the medicinal properties of thousands of substances, and understanding the effects obtained through the combination of these substances. Medicinal substances administered are not geared to eradicating symptoms, but to correcting the imbalance that brought those symptoms about.

According to the Tibetan scriptures, every natural substance in the world, animal, vegetable and mineral, can be used as medicine. Even deadly poisons may be transformed according to special procedures and used in medical formulas. The preparation of medicines is always accompanied by prayers that they be ultimately beneficial.

Tibetan medicine investigates illness according to a complex set of factors, many of which are not currently recognized or understood in the West. For instance, according to the Tibetan system, three cases of what we consider to be one disease (three cases of tuberculosis, for instance, or three cases of skin cancer) may be treated entirely differently, according to the particular imbalance which is perceived as having caused the disease. Prescribed treatments for what Westerners consider one disease might range widely; but each treatment is likely to include medicines made of herbs and other natural ingredients, modifications in diet, perhaps environmental changes and, for the Buddhist, contemplative practices or ritual.

According to the Tibetan medical texts, diseases have external (environmental), internal (dietary and behavior-related), and alternate or "secret" (psychological-spiritual) causes. Thus, Tibetan medicine involves a synthesis of physical, behavioral and psychological health practices. In prescribing a treatment, the physician considers many aspects of a patient's character and situation, including the patient's attitudes, behaviors, physical constitution, diet and home and work environments.

Following a strict, traditional approach to disease treatment, an imbalance is first treated with the most "gentle" of therapies, ranging from modifications in environment, diet and behavior to the inhalation of incense, bodily anointings, and herbal baths. Emetic-cathartic cleansings, medicines, and other physical therapies including moxibustion and acupuncture are added to treatment in cases of more extreme imbalance. Minor surgery and cauterization are considered radical forms of medicine, resorted to rarely.

Psychological-spiritual methods, including ritual and special contemplative practices, may be advised as accompaniment to all medical treatment, or they may be used alone. From a Tibetan

perspective, poor attitude and wrong behavior are two major contributors to imbalanced conditions in the body. A negative mental state will aggravate any physical disorder and diminish the value
of even the most effective medical treatments.

As the desired outcome of Tibetan medicine is always that of
balance, natural medicinal agents are combined and prepared in
special ways in order to encourage a state of physical and psychological equilibrium without harming the body in any way. Even
in highly acute cases, which might seem to demand the most dangerous drugs, Tibetan physicians carefully blend medical ingredients so that no one agent will shock the body or cause side effects
while "balancing" the body's chemistry.

Tibetan medicine today is evolving in response to the challenge
of new diseases such as AIDS and cancer. According to one Tibetan doctor who has toured the West extensively, "If a disease can
be understood, it can be treated.... With an understanding of any
disease, new treatments can be formulated." Accordingly, based on
information and formulas described in the ancient texts, new substances are being developed in keeping with doctors' observations
and experiences.

All Tibetan medical substances are made of natural ingredients:
minerals and metals, roots, flowers, leaves, fruits, seeds, tree bark
and sap, and animal products. In general, Tibetan doctors have
expressed concern about degenerating environmental conditions,
and call for a return to natural food products and a lowered use
of chemicals in our diet and environment, from food additives to
fertilizers, pesticides and nuclear waste.

Elements & Humors

Basic to Tibetan medical theory is the idea that the world and
everything in it is composed of combinations of the five
elements[2] wood, fire, earth, iron, water. Each of the elements has
a sympathetic and opposing relationship to other elements. A complex system of elemental relationships is reflected in every state
of matter, and in every condition of health or illness.[3]

The organs of the body are associated with and are specifically
affected by certain elements. For example, the liver and gallbladder are associated with the wood element; the heart and small intestine, with fire; the stomach and spleen with earth; the lungs
and large intestine with iron; the kidneys, reproductive vessels, and
bladder with water. Each season of the year is also associated with

a particular element.

In the human body, health reflects a balanced state of elemental relationships. Perceived through a thorough system of diagnosis, imbalance is corrected by natural medicinal substances, dietary support, and special practices in accordance with the time of year as well as the age, gender, and general character of the patient.

The five elements interact and combine to manifest in our bodies as three "humors" or principles of energy: wind, bile and phlegm. These humors affect and determine the physical and psychological qualities of a person. Although translations have rendered the names of the three humors as "wind, bile and phlegm," these words in Tibetan denote far more than their literal translations suggest.

The wind humor, although referring to more than what we think of as "breath," is directly related to breathing, nerve impulses, all movement throughout the body, the skeletal system, the organs of excretion and reproduction, the ears, and, on a psychological/spiritual level, awareness and knowing. In *Healing Herbs, The Heart of Tibetan Medicine*, by Badmajew, Badmajew and Park, the wind humor is described as an "intercom, receiving and sending messages between the organism and space.... representing physical and physiological motion."

The bile humor is primarily associated with fire and digestive heat. Because of bile's ability to extract nutrients from digested food and distribute these nutrients throughout the body, this humor is associated with the vascular system, the liver, and small intestines. Bile is also associated with the muscles, sight, skin, and the endocrine glands. Bile influences self-control and related aspects of intelligence.

The phlegm humor is a combination of earth and water elements. It is primarily associated with the lymphatic system, the mucous and serous membranes, the stomach, lungs, brain, and organs of taste and smell. Phlegm also affects one's ability to conceive children, to love, and to sleep, as well as one's capacity for compassion and wise judgment.

Every natural substance represents a unique combination of elements, and thus has a unique and specific effect upon humoral imbalances. The elemental combination characterizing any substance and its potential effects may be revealed through taste.

There are six basic tastes. A sweet taste results from a combination of the earth and water elements. Sour taste results from a combination of earth and fire elements. Salty taste results from the combination of water and fire. Bitter taste, from water and wind. A hot or acrid taste results from the combination of fire and air.

Astringent taste, from earth and wind together. Thus, in treating a patient, the physician prescribes herbal medicines or other substances, including everyday foods, according to the particular combination of elements, and thus medicinal qualities, of each substance. A sweet taste (earth and water) indicates an ability to subdue diseases of wind and bile. Substances characterized by sour (earth and fire), salty (water and fire), and burning or acrid (fire and air) tastes all have subduing effects on diseases of wind and phlegm. Bitter (water and air) and astringent (earth and air) tastes indicate a subduing effect upon bile disorders.

Although there are three humors, each humor is divided into five "branches." Thus there are fifteen basic humoral aspects, and fifteen categories of humoral activity. Each branch of the three humors has a direct connection with one aspect of physiology. For instance, examining the branches of the wind humor, we see that the "life-support wind," associated with the head and chest area, enables us to swallow, burp and sneeze. It is also associated with our sense organs and basic mental activities. The "ascending wind," functioning in the area of the nose, throat and tongue, governs our ability to speak, remember and pay attention. A malfunctioning "life-support wind" would cause disturbances to one's memory, speech, and ability to concentrate. The "all-pervading wind," which radiates from the body's center—the heart—to all parts of the body, regulates blood pressure and muscular activity. The "fire-accompanying wind," located in the lower stomach and large intestine, works directly to help the metabolism and digestion. This hot wind works in conjunction with the digestive bile to help insure proper assimilation of food and create healthy blood. Indigestion reflects a malfunctioning "fire-accompanying wind." Finally, the "downwards-voiding wind" is located in the area of the reproductive and excretory organs. It controls the release of sexual fluids as well as feces and urine.

The five "biles" and five "phlegms" are, likewise, each associated with specific organs and normal bodily functions as well as difficulties and disorders.

Every medicinal substance then, food included, is chosen for the combination of elements which make it up, and for the specific ways in which its particular combination of elements will affect the humoral nature of both patient and disease.

According to Tibetan Buddhist philosophy, the primary cause of all imbalance is our failure to recognize the oneness of all things—our insistence upon seeing ourselves as separate from all others. This dualistic division of the world into "self and other" is the source of what Buddhists call the three poisons: attachment, hatred and delusion. Each one of these poisons is related to one of the humors. On the metaphysical level, attachment is related to the humor of wind. Hatred or anger is related to the humor of bile. Delusion or ignorance is related to the humor of phlegm. These are perceived as secret, psychological-spiritual causes of imbalances which lead to disease. For this reason, the conscious employment of qualities such as compassion and awareness may be called upon as part of one's medical treatment, depending upon one's specific humoral character and imbalance.

Diagnosis

The Tibetans use various means of clinical diagnosis including physical observation, conversation with the patient, sphygmology (pulse diagnosis), and urinalyis.

First, the doctor relies on information gained through observation of the patient's physical qualities, such as size, coloring, voice, physical gestures, and the color and texture of the patient's tongue. Then the doctor asks about symptoms in much the same way as a Western doctor does. Questions about the patient's background, daily habits and environment help the doctor to formulate an opinion about possible causes of the patient's illness. A full set of questions relating to each of the three humors will help the doctor perceive which of these is causing the problem.

Next, in a procedure related to Chinese and Ayurvedic practices, the doctor feels six sets of pulses along the radial artery of each wrist. Pulse diagnosis enables the physician to become sensitive to a complex interplay of elements and humors in the body. It is the most important diagnostic tool used by the Tibetan physician— an ancient, highly complex practice requiring many years of training.

Each of the doctor's fingertips is divided into left and right halves; each half reads the condition of a specific organ. The pulses are named for those organs. Thus there is a "liver" pulse, a "heart" pulse, a "kidney" pulse, etc. The pulses are analyzed in relation to the elements and organs associated with them. The pulses reveal how the elements are working together, while indicating the characteristics of any humoral imbalance. There is no one "correct" pulse, and each person's ideal set of pulses changes according to the seasons and other environmental factors.

Urine evaluation is another important aspect of diagnosis. The color, texture and other qualities of the urine are analyzed to support or modify the doctor's conclusion about the patient's condition. Traditionally, urine is analyzed three times. When fresh, it is checked for color, steam, smell, and the quality of its bubbles or froth. When it is lukewarm, the albumin and oily chyle are analyzed. Finally, when the urine has cooled completely, it is checked for other variables.

According to ancient Tibetan texts, traditional methods of diagnosis are capable of revealing 84,000 states of imbalance. These imbalances are traditionally broken down to 1,616 ailments, then to 404 ailments, then to 101 major illnesses. These numerous conditions are generally treated according to guidelines established for fifteen types of humoral conditions: illnesses of the five winds, the five biles, and the five phlegms. But even these categories can be simplified further. On the most basic and important level, there are two kinds of diseases: those caused by heat and those caused by cold.

Accordingly, the first and most important thing a doctor must determine is whether an ailment is caused by overheating or overcooling in the body. A physician who has not made this distinction could harm a patient. According to Dr. Phuntsok Wangyal of the Tibetan Medical Institute in Dharamsala, India, applying a warming remedy to a heat-caused disease is very dangerous, like "setting fire to a dry tree." It may increase inflammation and other symptoms, while adding to the disease's ability to spread. Likewise, applying cooling substances to a patient suffering from a "cold" disease will most likely cause that disease to worsen and spread.

Cancer

As we know, Western medicine categorizes cancer as essentially one disease which manifests in many different ways. From the perspective of Tibetan medicine, however, every case of cancer is caused by a specific and individualized elemental imbalance. Some cancers may emerge as the result of a wind imbalance. Others may be brought on through disturbed bile or phlegm. Treatment is always administered according to the source of the imbalance. A cancer caused by a disorder of bile (excessive heat or fire element in the body) will generally be treated by foods and medicines with cooling properties. Cancers caused by a disorder of phlegm (excessive earth and water elements in the body) or wind (excessive air) will be treated by foods and medicines with warming qualities.

In treating cancer, it is especially essential that proper diagnosis has been made in terms of the disease's hot or cold nature. A hot-natured cancer, if not controlled, may ripen and burst, causing a fatal metastasis. A cold-natured cancer, in contact with cold-producing foods and medicines, will also be encouraged to grow and, eventually, to metastasize.

All cancer medicines are specially blended for the individual condition. Primary components are always accompanied by modifying subcomponents in order to strengthen the organ or organs involved while weakening the cancer. Even in the most serious cases, care is taken to avoid all side effects or other damages to the body.

Consistent with the Tibetan belief that each cancer is caused by a unique interplay of elements and environmental conditions, cancer medicines vary greatly, according to the particular type of imbalance suffered by the cancer patient. Although certain ingredients are common to many medicines used in cancer treatment, there is no one "cancer medicine." The Tibetan physician works with all the information made available through diagnosis in order to most effectively "stimulate some elements and subdue others."

Tibetan physicians want to encourage their patients' own ability to recover psychological and physical balance. Even when facing life-threatening cancers, they strive to cooperate with the patient's own system. Highly invasive treatments such as surgery and radiation are rarely, if ever, employed; cytotoxic chemotherapy is never employed. The Tibetans believe that such methods interfere with the patient's own life-energy pathways, and, thus, with the healing process itself.

As far as extant records suggest, what we call "cancer" today was very rare in Tibet prior to the Chinese occupation in 1959. People did get tumors, but when imbalances were identified, cures were effected through the traditional medical system. Relatively few tumors became cancerous. Tibetan doctors have hypothesized that the increase of cancer in the West and even in places like India is greatly due to environmental pollution in many forms, and further affected by the fear and depression which so often accompany the knowledge that one has the "dreaded" disease. These emotions are said to literally depress the body's ability to balance itself.

Cancers are considered to be "nyen," a specific type of disease especially prevalent in the modern age. "Nyen" diseases are perceived as the fruit of a combination of environmental (external), nutritional-behavioral (internal), psychological-spiritual (alternate or "secret") imbalances, and other conditions which characterize our time.

External causes of cancer include the pollution of our air, water, earth, and other aspects of our environment. On the physical level, it is poison which causes cancer, but poison is not strictly limited to the physical realm.

Internal causes of cancer may include chronic indigestion, a state which is often stimulated by poor food-combining as well as by improper mental outlook while eating. Poor digestion contributes directly to the internal cause of cancer, believed to be "weakened blood." According to the Tibetan system, blood influences the strength of our organs, and its weakened state is deemed responsible for many modern diseases.

One cause of poor digestion and weakened blood is a lack of heat in the stomach. Drinking and eating extremely cold things can destroy the stomach's digestive heat and may contribute to "weakened blood." Highly refined and sweet foods, composed primarily of the earth and water elements, have the same effect. If digestion is impaired, the pure essence of food is not transformed into blood. This may cause the development of cancerous and non-cancerous tumors, water-related imbalances, and ulcer-like conditions.

Once a cancer is present, it is greatly exaggerated by the consumption of "extreme" foods such as alchohol, beef, pork, garlic and onions, strong tea and coffee, dairy products, sugar, sour foods and beverages. Such foods encourage wind-energy disturbances, and thus, a spreading of the cancer throughout the body.

Wind energy, responsible for all circulation, is considered to be the source of cancer's ability to spread. Once this process has begun, the Tibetan doctor will try to keep the wind energy from increasing, while working to stop any inflammation of the tumor, which is associated with heat. Food and drink, such as alcohol and meat, which cause a heating effect must be strictly avoided. Some tumors may be cauterized as a means of cutting them off from the rest of the blood and from nutrients carried by the blood. In most cases, medicine is given to stop the ripening of the tumor, and also to bring the wind energy down to a balanced, stabilized state. As wind energy is also related with activity of the mind, it is considered important that the cancer patient seek moderation in mental as well as physical activity.

Alternate or *"secret"* causes of diseases such as cancer involve subtle, unconscious thought processes. Negative thinking is believed to stimulate illness. Secret causes may include modern-day frustrations and stress, as well as what we call "repression" or other psychological blocks and imbalances. Thoughts or "patterns of mind" influence the wind patterns in the passages of the body. The wind patterns themselves influence the quality of energy in the body, which can either strengthen or weaken the body's resistance to disease. Mind, then, is seen as an intrinsic influence upon all states of physical well-being or illness.

Once a person has cancer, the Tibetan doctor stresses the need to maintain a positive emotional outlook. A patient who can relate to his or her situation and accept spiritual advice, is considered to be in a good position for healing, which may take place on the physical and/or spiritual level.

Cancer Prevention

While external causes of disease may include pollution and the use of chemicals, internal and secret factors include aspects of our behavior and our emotions. So Tibetan physicians suggest that we reduce the likelihood of getting cancer by seeking moderation and avoiding aggression, on both physical and mental levels. It is recommended that one breathe clean air and eat natural food that has not been poisoned by chemicals such as human-made fertilizers and pesticides. While a wholesome environment and a relaxed mind can be the most important factors in preventing many cancers, foods producing extreme heat—including spices, alcoholic beverages, beef and pork; and extreme cold—cold drinks, sweet and refined food products—should be avoided as well.

Based on ancient medical texts, the Tibetans have developed a formula which is used for both prevention and treatment of many cancerous conditions. This formula, which calls for detoxified mercury, minerals and metals including gold, silver and zinc, is shaped into pill form. Its use as a universal antidote, rejuvenating agent, and disease-prevention treatment makes the "precious pill" or Jewel Medicine a highly revered commodity in China, Tibet, India and by some today in the U.S.

In Bhopal, India, during the emergency caused by widespread exposure to toxic chemicals in 1984, nearly three hundred Tibetans were exposed to the poisonous fumes. Since most Tibetans take one or two "precious pills" wherever they go, the medicine was distributed among Tibetans in the vicinity of the accident. The pills were so effective that when the Tibetans came in contact with the poison, they immediately started eliminating it. None of the Tibetans died. Many requests for the pills were made, and hundreds were sent to Bhopal specifically for use by the Indian people.

Prophecies on Cancer

Ancient Tibetan prophecies have alluded to the occurrence of cancer and other modern diseases during an era which may seem, upon reflection, somewhat like our own.

Gyu-zhi, the primary medical text of Tibet, records prophecies made by author Yuthok Yonten Gompo I, a scholar and sage believed to have possessed the qualities of the Medicine Buddha. These prophecies, made in the eighth century A.D., tell of a future wherein humans are highly confused. Production and consumption of material goods are described as being the main thing on these people's minds, and so they are tremendously busy, always trying to be productive. But their confusion, or their inability to see what is truly needed for the benefit of all life on the planet, causes them to produce many "evil artificial substances" which actually poison them. These poisons, in the water, in the air, in the earth, and in their food, are prophesied as being the external cause of much illness (and contributing to the internal cause); the alternate or secret causes of these illnesses being excessive attachment, hatred, and delusion or ignorance.

Yuthok Yonten Gompo I also taught that the humans of that future time would be in delicate state of environmental and internal imbalance. Radical or violent means of medical intervention, such as strong chemical medicines, would throw their systems into total disorder. So as to avoid this in any age, gentle, supportive and strengthening methods of healing form the basic Tibetan approach to medicine.

One prophecy recorded in the *Gyu-zhi* mentions a category of disease attributed to great technological development and ensuing environmental pollution. This "nyen" category of disease, to which cancer belongs, is described as becoming prominent at a time of much movement and upheaval in the earth, a time of much excavation and activity, from mining to building in the environment. Places characterized by such activity are described as being the most likely places for people to get cancer and related diseases. People's minds are described as being far less relaxed during that time and much more busily involved in the world, their careers and related activities. Depression, mental tension, and high intake of alcohol all contribute to the "nyen" diseases, which are caused most directly, on a physical level, by the contamination of substances in our environment.

The emergence of cancer and other epidemic diseases during this time of increased chemical use makes these imbalances worthy of a special category. They are not considered to be diseases of individual karma (caused by the thoughts and deeds of individuals during this or past lifetimes). Instead, getting such diseases may be seen as the fruit of deeds and thought patterns which are shared by a great many people of this age.

Spiritual Medicine

In traditional Tibetan society, the relationship between medicine and Buddhist philosophy is so close that many practicing physicians are actually lamas or priests as well. Medical doctors are held in high esteem, second only to the lamas.

Traditional Tibetan doctors integrate the philosophy and spiritual discipline of Buddhism with the mechanical aspects of their work. They pray and practice specific healing rituals daily in order to be open to the all-pervading knowledge and power of the Medicine Buddha; and to take on the Buddha's virtuous qualities, especially his great and shining compassion. This compassion radiates to those who are receptive to it, and helps to eliminate the three mental "poisons" (attachment, hatred and ignorance) which, according to Buddhism, are secret contributing factors to physical illness. Meritorious practices including contemplative activity and the making of ritual offerings are advised for all those who would like to increase their intuitive contact with the power of the Medicine Buddha.

The Medicine Buddha is invoked during all phases of the doctor's work, including herb-gathering, medicine-compounding, and one-to-one counseling. The potency of every Tibetan medicine is considered to come from both its physical ingredients and the quality of care and loving kindness expressed by the person involved in the collecting, compounding, and application of that medicine. The doctor's selfless intention to benefit beings, the sonic vibrations of the doctor's invocations to the Medicine Buddha through recitation of mantras and prayers, and the thoughtful and delicate nature of the doctor's or pharmacist's approach to the medicine-making process, all have an effect on the medicine. A good rap-

port between doctor and patient allows the patient to feel the healing quality of the Medicine Buddha as it manifests through the
doctor, and ultimately helps to make any treatment most beneficial.

Healing depends upon effective "seeing" with a healing intent
by both doctor and patient. The patient often participates actively in the healing process through visualizations, which might include seeing the doctor embodying the qualities of the Medicine
Buddha. The doctor may also visualize the patient as being filled
with light. Many Westerners who have been treated by Tibetan
doctors, even those who have never heard of the Medicine Buddha or practiced special visualization techniques, have experienced
the physical healing effects of Tibetan medicine, and consistently
tell of an unusual "kindness" emanating from the doctors who have
treated them.

The quality of the relationship between the doctor and the patient has a strong effect upon the outcome of an illness. Medicines
are considered to be far more effective if the patient has faith or
trust in the doctor. According to Tibetan Buddhism, the doctor-
patient relationship is greatly affected by the spiritual practice and
virtuous activities of both individuals.

A patient who does not respond to normal medical treatment
may be experiencing what is sometimes called karmic or "evolutionary illness" caused by deeds of the past. If a disease is deemed
to be of an evolutionary nature, a medical cure is not pursued. Instead, the patient is confronted with the idea that such disease
may not be curable by physical means because of his or her own
personal stage of spiritual development. The doctor then exposes
that patient to intensive spiritual teachings, and recommends that
the patient receive blessings and practice certain meditations, re-
cite certain prayers or mantras, and make special offerings. The
physician's wish, in this case, is not primarily that the patient be
physically saved, but that the patient will be able to turn that im-
minent death into growth or progress on the spiritual path.

Interestingly, the ritual treatment itself may have a radical effect
on some diseases. Certain patients have overcome psychological
and physical obstacles through spiritual practice alone.

According to Tibetan Buddhist philosophy, one function of all
disease is to stimulate compassionate activity. If a patient meditates on compassion, benefits will be sensed on both physical and
psychological levels. The Tibetans believe that a compassionate
person with a relaxed state of mind will enjoy stable, balanced energy, and will accumulate great merit on the spiritual plane.

So convinced are Tibetan physicians of the value of spiritual prac-

tices in treating disease that several have expressed interest in seeing the results of Western, double-blind experiments comparing
the results of medical treatment on pairs of patients with similar
physical conditions. Their suggestion is that one member of each
pair be a serious practitioner of a spiritual discipline, the other member of each pair (part of the control group), not a practitioner.

Tibetan Medicine & Astrology

Five-element theory is the first point of relationship between
Tibetan medicine and astrology. The parts of the body, directions,
and hours of the day are all ruled by specific elements. Tibetan
doctors are well aware of the relationship among the humors, time
of day, and the season. For instance, someone suffering from a wind-
energy disturbance due to tension and stress will feel far worse
at night (and during hot, rainy weather), and may suffer from in-
somnia. Someone suffering from a hot-natured, bile-related condition will suffer more between noon and midnight (and during
warm, post-rainy weather). A cold-natured, phlegm-related condition will cause one to suffer more during early morning (and during the late winter). Medicine, then, will often be prescribed for
the morning, and/or afternoon, and/or evening. A hot-natured
medicine will be given in the morning in order to build up a little
heat in the system and subdue a phlegmatic condition. Medicines
given during the afternoon are cooler-natured compounds which
will subdue bile-related disorders. Medicines given at night help
one to relax, to sleep better, to help stabilize the wind energy. The
astrologer also works with a network of protective spirits, each rul-
ing over a particular time of year. He may encourage patients to
make special offerings or otherwise become more mindful of the
qualities represented by each of these spirits.

Astrologers often work in tandem with medical doctors to establish balance among the elements for patients. For instance, the
Tibetan astrologer may calculate the location of the patient's "aperture of la"[4] and advise the physician as to the timeliness of certain treatments such as moxibustion, acupuncture or surgery.

The astrologer may also complement the physician's work by
recommending and/or performing rituals which emphasize the relationship between the patient's special elemental make-up/im-
balance and the environment. For instance, if a patient is deficient
in the wood element, the astrologer may supplement the doctor's
recommendations by advising the patient to plant and care for a

tree facing in an appropriate direction. Such activities are believed to have a focusing and healing effect on the mind of the patient.

East-West Exchange

Over 2,500 years ago, the historical Buddha Sakyamuni taught of the atom and even of infinitely more subtle subatomic particles. Although microscopes and other sophisticated scientific equipment were not used in Tibet before 1959, the Tibetan scientific tradition offers information, techniques, and new perspectives which potentially complement Western science. Many Tibetan doctors await the Western discovery of various subatomic particles which are discussed in the ancient *Kalachakra* (Wheel of Time) *Tantra*, a text which describes our relationship with time and space.

In spite of a lack of communication between Tibetan and Western scientists, greatly due to centuries of geographical isolation as well as linguistic and ideological differences, intercultural dialogue is being advanced at universities, medical centers, research foundations, and Buddhist teaching centers throughout the world. This dialogue, and its results, have the potential to benefit people everywhere.

For example, although surgery (except for cataract removal and certain drainage procedures) is generally not practiced by traditional Tibetan doctors today[5], certain Tibetan procedures may support Western surgical practices. For instance, since the Tibetans believe that surgery may cause the "roots" of a tumor to spread, it is recommended that the tumors themselves be treated before surgery with medicines or cauterization in order to encourage them to shrink and retreat from their surroundings. These and other methods could be used in the West to make surgery and other practices more effective and recovery more comfortable.

Certainly, the merging of ancient Tibetan philosophy and practices with the benefits of modern Western resources and technology represents a union of tremendous potential. Going beyond the limitations of both systems, such a collaboration will contribute to the creation of an optimum model of medicine: broad, flexible, effective, and answering the needs of human beings on physical, behavioral and psychological-spiritual levels.

Afterword

This chapter has been compiled from extensive interviews on

the science of Tibetan medicine with Dr. Tenzin Chudrak, Dr. Phuntsok Wangyal, Dr. Trogawa Rinpoche, Dr. Lobsang Drolma, a taped lecture on cancer by Dr. Yeshi Donden, and several articles, books and pamphlets. Special thanks as well to Chinese astrologer Dr. Jin Shiang Shiah.

In spite of our efforts to westernize the presentation of this ancient Oriental culture, I am committed to the idea that the Tibetan system, like all systems, be studied and understood in the context of its own origin and practice. I encourage further study, and recommend the following publications:

Tibetan Medicine Series: journals published by the Library of Tibetan Works and Archives, Dharamsala, India, 1980 - present.

Health Through Balance by Dr. Yeshi Donden, ed. and tr. by Jeffrey Hopkins. Snow Lion Publications, Ithaca, New York 1986.

Tibetan Medicine: a Holistic Approach to Better Health by Dr. Lobsang Rapgay, Ph.D. Dr. Lobsang Rapgay, Dharamsala, India, 1984.

Tibetan Buddhist Medicine and Psychiatry: the Diamond Healing by Terry Clifford. Samuel Weiser, Inc., York Beach, Maine, 1983.

Healing Herbs: the Heart of Tibetan Medicine by Pater Badmajew, Jr., M.D., Vladimir Badmajew, Jr., M.D., Lynn Park. Red Lotus Press, Berkeley, California 1982.

Fundamentals of Tibetan Medicine According to the Rgyud-Bzhi by T.J. Tsarong. Tibetan Medical Centre, Dharamsala, India 1981.

The Ambrosia Heart Tantra: the Secret Oral Teaching on the Eight Branches of the Science of Healing by Dr. Yeshi Donden, tr. by Jhampa Kelsang. Library of Tibetan Works and Archives, Dharamsala, India 1977.

Tibetan Medicine by the Venerable Rechung Rinpoche, tr. by Jampal Kunzang. University of California Press, Berkeley and Los Angeles, California 1973.

Notes

1. The word "astrology" is actually a loose translation. The "science of time and space" is far removed from the astrology familiar to Westerners. In the Tibetan tradition, medicine and the science of time and space are based on many of the same principles, and are very closely related. Every Tibetan doctor has done

some study in the field of astrology, which is based on the ancient Chinese system as well as the *Kalachakra* system believed to have been taught by the Buddha in India in 600 B.C.; and every astrologer has studied medicine. In Tibetan culture, religion, medicine, and astrology are interrelated aspects of one central science.

Tibetan astrologers are scholars of several disciplines, including Sanskrit language and poetics, indispensable in deciphering and applying relevant ancient texts. The astrologer, according to the patterns shown in a person's astrological chart, may advise a particular type of community service in order to change the individual's karma. Rituals, special behaviors and diet will be recommended; the astrologer may advise one to avoid certain foods or certain emotions; he or she may advise little or no travel, or a certain kind of work. All of the astrologer's recommendations are based on the tradition of Indo-Tibetan Buddhist practice. Often these practices are designed to complement medical treatment.

Both the Tibetan medical and astrological systems stress training of the mind. Tibetan physicians and astrologers believe that anything can be created by the mind and one's way of seeing. The concept that karma can be affected through virtuous action and mind training is integral to Tibetan Buddhist culture, and reflects the hope that much of the energy on our planet may be balanced.

2. Two sets of "five elements" are used in the Tibetan medical system. One, associated primarily with philosophical aspects of Tibetan science, originated in India as part of the Ayurvedic system. It is comprised of earth, fire, water, air and space. Also referred to in Tibetan Medicine are the five elements derived from the Chinese astrological system: wood, fire, earth, iron, water. These have a more common, practical application, and are of primary value in the practices of diagnosis, prescription and divination.

3. Each element is said to be the source or "mother" of another, the friend of another, and the antagonist or "foe" of yet another. The diagram on page 264 shows these relationships. Vertically, from the top, we see that wood is the mother of fire; fire is the "son" of wood. Fire is the mother of earth; earth the son of fire. Earth is the mother of iron; iron is the son of earth. Iron is the mother of water; water is the son of iron. Water is the mother of wood, and wood is the son of water.

The mother-son relationship reflects an ongoing creative cycle, through which one element creates another. For instance, wood feeds fire, and the ashes which are produced become part of the earth. The earth's pressure creates metal, which in turn produces water, which gives life to vegetation (wood).

Friend-foe relationships are a bit more complex, and may seem paradoxical. For instance, starting horizontally from the left, the enemy of fire is water; and yet the friend of water is fire. The enemy of water is earth, yet the friend of earth is water. The enemy of earth is wood; the friend of wood is earth. The enemy of wood is iron; the friend of iron is wood. The enemy of iron is fire; the friend of fire is iron.

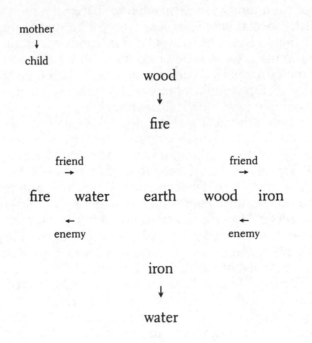

4. The "brightness" of one's "la," the natural energy quality of an individual, is a function of wind energy which greatly affects one's life expectancy. The "aperture of la" moves throughout the body in a monthly cycle, and the piercing or injury of that aperture is highly dangerous.

5. Tibet does have a tradition of surgical practice, but it was discontinued during the eighth century due to the death of a noblewoman following unsuccessful surgery.

Epilogue

Along with the reality of cancer in our time, two themes have been woven through this book. The first is consciousness, specifically a consciousness that effects healing. The second is the importance of dialogue as a means of expanding and activating that consciousness.

Much of the intercultural dialogue presented in this work takes place through the voices of medical doctors, scientists and philosophers of Tibet and the modern West. I do not equate post-industrial society with the West, nor is Tibet meant to represent the East. Simply put, these are the two cultures which I know, and from which I have learned so much.

Prior to writing this book, I had studied Tibetan Buddhist meditation and iconography for two decades. But through the purposeful pursuit of dialogue on cancer, I achieved a new level of understanding of the Buddha's own teaching that dualistic thought and action—which create the illusion of separate realities like "self" and "other"—are the source of all suffering. We are a part of nature; if we continue to see ourselves as separate from nature, as its "conquerers," we, the citizens of planet Earth, will not only pay the price of increased suffering—we simply may not survive.

In line with the Buddha's teachings in 600 BC, post-Einsteinian physical scientists have observed that every particle of matter is related to and actually affects every other particle in the universe. Clearly, all who are alive today and sharing this planet are closely related and interdependent.

Through an accelerated process of mechanization and industrialization, we have experienced a decline in many of the universal

265

values and systems which have supported human life in relationship with the Earth for thousands of years. We put immediate satisfaction and gain before ecological balance, and ignore what many Native American peoples regard as the need to "accept or reject technology based upon how it will affect the survival of seven generations into the future." Thus we are living with the results of a technology which has polluted our air, water, and soil. Even our food chain has been extensively contaminated with harmful chemical additives and "preservative" radiation. An industrial approach which puts manufacturers' convenience and profit before nutrition and long-term health literally threatens our survival.

We have arrived at a point of crisis in both physical and mental health care, systems which depend greatly upon our modern technology. Now we must reclaim many of the values that we have lost, and we have a great deal to learn from ancient cultures. For while when our modern industrial and post-industrial technology (not even two centuries old) threatens all life on this planet, ancient cultures' adherence to tradition has enabled them to survive for thousands of years and longer. There is no need to reinvent the wheel; but there *is* a great need to investigate and learn from others as we draw upon the wisdom of our ancestors. This is key as we work toward resolving many of the challenges which we face today.

On the medical front, specialization has contributed to the isolation of various fields. The realms of gynecology, cardiology and psychology, for example, are regarded by many practitioners as independent areas of study and treatment. This situation has contributed to the development of medicines which, while causing certain positive therapeutic effects, may compromise the immune system and otherwise injure the body as a whole.

Today's trend toward complementary medicine and the science of psychoneuroimmunology—described by some as the newest medical science—brings us full circle to the knowledge and wisdom of traditional cultures which recognize the intrinsic relationship and interdependence among all parts of the whole human being and between human beings and our environment. Ironically perhaps, this recognition in modern society may be a direct result of the kinds of diseases we are now suffering. (Both cancer and AIDS affect the immune system, causing generalized states of weakness and vulnerability.)

Just as we are redeveloping an awareness of the importance of nutrition and a healthy environment, we are also coming to recognize the effects of psychological states ranging from stress to deep relaxation on our physical well being. Millions of cancer and AIDS patients have discovered that psychic healing methods plus community support can enrich and even extend their lives. Thus, we rediscover that the purpose of medicine may very well be to strengthen the entire organism, not just to eliminate certain symptoms which keep the person from performing normally in society. Today, through a synthesis of ancient and new technologies, we may effect true healing on many levels.

For more than a thousand years in Buddhist Tibet, physicians have prayed that their motivation be pure and unselfish, and that the blessings and essence of the Medicine Buddha be bestowed upon them before beginning to work with each patient. The patient is aware of this, and recognizes the medical practitioner as having embodied the Buddha's healing qualities and abilities. In Tibetan culture, the relationship between physician and patient is considered to be extremely important in the resolution of both mental and physical imbalance.

And we in the post-industrial West are approaching similar themes in interesting ways. In dialogues ranging from that with radiologist Dr. Seymour Brenner to one with master of macrobiotic theory and practice Michio Kushi, the success of a treatment is linked to patient's conscious involvement in the healing process, whether through dietary adjustments or changes in consciousness or attitude.

This growing awareness is extremely important in our time, for in having lost our sense of vital relationship with nature, so have we lost a trust in our own intuitive perceptions of what is going on within our own bodies and psyches. According to one doctor, the denial of our own bodily messages is one of the reasons that so many cancer patients only discover their disease when it is far too late.

Meanwhile, the tremendous role of consciousness (otherwise known as "psychological elements") in the healing process is being celebrated in such books as Dr. Bernie Siegel's *Love, Medicine and Miracles*. This book's continuing popularity reflects our eagerness to re-learn the ways through which emotional and spiritual growth can effect healing.

The Dalai Lama has stated that consciousness can only be understood through consciousness, and that it is through the study of consciousness that we may come to understand and learn to deal with matter. Today's physicists postulate that matter can be affected and even created through consciousness.

Indeed, cancer cells have been known to retreat like a virus when treated like a virus, to respond to metabolic adjustment when treated as metabolic imbalance, to retreat in response to dietary changes, meditation, cell-killing chemotherapy, radiation and many other forms of intervention.

We might conclude that each treatment reacts biophysically and chemically in a unique way with each cancer, depending upon the whole physical and psychological chemistry of the person being treated in the context of her or his environment. We can observe attitude affecting reality on another level when we see how perceptions such as "it's survival of the fittest" and "all for the common good" each affect social organization, patterns of relationship — and as discussed by Dr. Dwight McKee, even medical practice.

Through years of meditation on the notion of impermanence, I have come to realize that we are on this Earth to protect and nurture the evolution of consciousness. Activation of this attitude will enable us to discover and develop new ways of warming our homes, putting food on the table, bringing us the news, and moving ahead through the next generations in peace and abundance. We have a tremendous amount of learning to do, learning which calls for flexibility and great creativity as we design a future of renewable resources and medicines that heal as they nourish and strengthen. This can only come about through the harnessing of ancient as well as modern technologies in ways that exploit no one but serve us all.

Surely, this goal can be reached through dialogue. We must aspire to a consciousness that enables us to share and exchange diverse and sometimes conflicting points of view with one another, a consciousness that enables us to transform a deadly and dreaded disease into a teacher and even an ally, a consciousness that enables us to imagine and finally create a technology of healing, one which encourages the innate power of each organism to heal itself.

I imagine a place that physical scientists, scientists of the mind and spirit, scientists of all persuasions and cultures might visit for days, months, years at a time... not in service to any particular government or personal gain, but for the good of all humanity and future generations of humanity. For as we recognize our need for dialogue and a healing consciousness, this is the leadership we need, motivated by the pure intent to benefit all beings, including our planet.

DEDICATION OF MERIT

On both individual and societal levels, we can no longer ask our selves, "What is best for me?" Our connection to all living things must motivate us to ask always, "What attitudes, actions, and technologies benefit all, including our planet?" May we generate this benefit by answering and acting upon questions like "How can I be a part of this?"

INDEX

271

SIGO PRESS

SIGO PRESS publishes books in psychology which continue the work of C.G. Jung, the great Swiss psychoanalyst and founder of analytical psychology. Each season SIGO brings out a small but distinctive list of titles intended to make a lasting contribution to psychology and human thought. These books are invaluable reading for Jungians, psychologists, students and scholars and provide enrichment and insight to general readers as well. In the Jungian Classics Series, well-known Jungian works are brought back into print in popular editions.

Other Titles from Sigo Press

The Unholy Bible *by June Singer*

Emotional Child Abuse *by Joel Covitz*

Dreams of a Woman *by Shelia Moon*

Androgyny *by June Singer*

The Dream-The Vision of the Night *by Max Zeller*

Sandplay Studies *by Bradway et al.*

Symbols Come Alive in the Sand *by Evelyn Dundas*

Inner World of Childhood *by Frances G. Wickes*

Inner World of Man *by Frances G. Wickes*

Inner World of Choice *by Frances G. Wickes*

Available from SIGO PRESS, 25 New Chardon Street, #8748A, Boston, Massachusetts, 02114. tel. (508) 526-7064

In England: Element Books, Ltd., Longmead, Shaftesbury, Dorset, SP7 8PL. tel. (0747) 51339, Shaftesbury.